BRAIN-
POWERED
WEIGHT
LOSS

BRAIN-POWERED WEIGHT LOSS

THE 11-STEP BEHAVIOR-BASED PLAN
THAT ENDS OVEREATING
AND LEADS TO DROPPING
UNWANTED POUNDS FOR GOOD

ELIZA KINGSFORD
WITH DEBORA YOST

RODALE.

613.25
KIN

1-9-17 ML

RODALE *wellness*

Live happy. Be healthy. Get inspired.

Sign up today to get exclusive access to our authors, exclusive bonuses,
and the most authoritative, useful, and cutting-edge information on health,
wellness, fitness, and living your life to the fullest.

Visit us online at RodaleWellness.com
Join us at RodaleWellness.com/Join

Book design by Amy King

Library of Congress Cataloging-in-Publication Data is on file with the Publisher.

ISBN-13: 978–1–62336–809–8 hardcover

Distributed to the trade by Macmillan

2   4   6   8   10   9   7   5   3   1   hardcover

 RODALE.

We inspire health, healing, happiness, and love in the world. Starting with you.

*To Tom, who is always pushing me
to do and be my best.*

*To all of the Wellspring families we've served over the years,
your courage is inspiring. I hope this offers you some wisdom
and support on your journey.*

CONTENTS

FOREWORD

Food, Behavior, Addiction, and Overweight

I have worked for more than 40 years trying to understand how food, sugar, and drugs of abuse hijack the brain, insinuate themselves into the users' thoughts, stimulate their own taking, and cause addictions. During this time, neuroscientists have made great progress in understanding where each drug of abuse goes in the brain and body and the changes that occur during intoxication and withdrawal. We can now pinpoint where in the brain the effects are taking place. This has opened new horizons, enabling us to approach the treatment of obesity in promising new ways.

A lot of progress has been made in our understanding of obesity since the days when we began to focus on the conditions associated with obesity, such as diabetes, heart disease, kidney disease, cancer, and joint problems, like we focused on the emphysema, bronchitis, cancers, and osteoporosis associated with smoking. We now have a new understanding for how bariatric surgery and pharmacological treatments work, and have seen the approval of new medications for obesity based on the addictive nature of certain foods. Still, these treatments are not cures, are incomplete, and work best in the context of a life-changing program. Putting research into clinical practice is quite complicated and is always a work in progress. It requires that someone take a concept or concepts, weave them into the matrix of a caring program, test outcomes, and adjust—while still helping to move the field forward.

I consider Eliza Kingsford a national leader in weight management. The reason: What the rest of us have discovered in academia, laboratory, and clinical settings, this pioneer has actually put into practice. The culmination of all her knowledge and successful hands-on experience in helping people find the solution to their weight-loss issues is the book you have in your hands.

Kingsford, a licensed psychotherapist, is the leader of Wellspring, the largest, oldest, and most-respected noninstitutional weight-loss program in the world. What she has achieved in her 10-year tenure, including two years as executive director, is nothing short of extraordinary. Rarely is an expert so grounded in science and the actual delivery of overweight and obesity treatment. Kingsford has learned by working with national and international experts, listening, and applying these insights in an open-air camp setting. She has worked with thousands of young people who have serious issues with food, including the stigma, shame, and trauma that often are part of it all. She knows and studies the literature and applies it in the field, ferreting out what doesn't work (or doesn't work very well), and polishing and improving what benefits people and helps them come to terms with their own food addictions and behaviors that drive their urge to overeat.

I have worked to understand food-brain reward and its relationship to drugs of abuse and addictions since the early 1980s. I am lucky to have worked with leading obesity and food addiction experts: the late Bart Hoebel, PhD, formerly of Princeton University; and Kelly D. Brownell, PhD, of Duke University and formerly of Yale; as well as other top food and addiction experts, including Nicole Avena, PhD; Ashley Gearhardt, PhD; Samuel Klein, MD; Louis J. Aronne, MD; Robert H. Lustig, MD; Gene-Jack Wang, MD; and Marc N. Potenza, MD. Yes, we have really found that, for many people, eating is an addiction as powerful as cigarettes, recreational drugs, gambling, and sex.

Failed diets and attempts to control overeating, preoccupation with food and eating, and the shame, anger, and guilt that follow look and respond like traditional addictions. It is common for people to overeat beyond fullness for the same brain reward that drives people to smoke, take recreation drugs, gamble, and engage in unhealthy sexual practices. These experts and I have been instrumental in helping Kingsford translate and advance our laboratory science into Wellspring's treatment program and the first-of-its kind do-it-yourself plan she created called Brain-Powered Weight Loss. Just as we use behavioral therapies to overcome these addictions, Kingsford uses the same and similar therapies to help people overcome the grip that food has on their day-to-day lives. It's the link that is missing from all other weight-related programs.

Eliza Kingsford gets it. She understands that the reason overweight and obese people behave in unhealthy ways around food, in spite of the potentially devastating consequences, is because they have a dysfunctional relationship with food. This is the reason why achieving *permanent* weight loss is so difficult. She also knows that it is possible to address the trauma, shame, stigma, and the effects of food, especially highly palatable food, on the brain. The most novel part of her plan is the tools she uses, which have little to do with what someone should or should not eat in order to lose weight. Her tools are all powered by the brain—self-implementing techniques, based on proven cognitive therapies, that help people change the way they think and behave around food.

What is more striking and impresses me the most about her successful approach is her goal to steer people toward better physical and mental health, balance, well-being, and wellness. I believe in her program—it will evolve as science and evidence change. It offers the most promise to people who are trying to overcome their struggle with overweight and obesity on their own.

Kingsford brings an innovative and unique approach to achieving long-term weight-loss success in a way that's almost unheard of: by teaching over-eaters how to change long-ingrained habits that drive an unhealthy relationship with food. Once you read this book, you'll find, as others have, that it is possible to calmly and assuredly be in control of your relationship with food instead of the other way around.

Mark S. Gold, MD
17th Distinguished Alumni Professor, University of Florida;
Adjunct Professor of Psychiatry, Washington University, St. Louis;
Chair, Scientific Advisory Boards for RiverMend Health, a national provider
of addiction, eating disorders, and obesity evaluation and treatment

WHY I WROTE THIS BOOK

For more than a decade, I have been helping people overcome their weight-loss issues. They usually end up in my office unhappy with their relationship with food and their bodies, and are ready to make a change.

What I've observed on a regular basis is a problem at the intersection of theory and practice. By that I mean people are buoyed when the newest diet book (theory) comes out, only to find themselves disappointed in the eventual outcome (practice). They know what they *should* do, what the latest science suggests, and what the latest research supports, yet they struggle with *why* they can't seem to make it work.

I've found that the key to success must involve both theory and practice. There is a need for both. We need to know what the science of weight loss is teaching us, but more so, we need to understand human behavior. Somehow, after reading all the latest diet books—many written by incredibly knowledgeable and talented doctors and scientists—people lose weight, only to go back to engaging in the same behaviors they had before the diet began. You know where that leads!

I am not saying that going on this or that plan can't work. Many diets out there can and do work temporarily, but it's not enough. They're too short-lived. That missing link called human behavior—our old habits and their relationship with our food choices—is the downfall of even the very best diets.

This is not to criticize the worth of healthy weight-loss plans and the intention of the people who create them. I am not a doctor or a scientist or a researcher as many of these experts are. I am a licensed therapist who specializes in weight loss. I have an immense amount of respect for the science that goes into writing these diet books. Some of the scientists, doctors, and researchers who author them are my mentors, my heroes, and certainly the people who guide my own work. I feel there is a need for everyone who is overweight to understand the science behind weight loss—what's good, what's not so good, what initiates weight gain, what promotes fat burn, and so on. There are thousands of studies and books supporting these theories, all valid aids that could probably solve most anyone's weight dilemma.

However, there is still that missing link. We need to get a grasp on the human behavior that drives weight gain. There is a need to understand the complex everyday emotions that drive our decisions around food, which have nothing to do with what we *know* about weight loss and everything to do with how we *feel* and *think* about food. This is the reason why this book came to be.

You will find *Brain-Powered Weight Loss* different from any diet you've ever tried or any diet book you've ever read. For starters, it is not a "diet" in the traditional sense. Yes, I do map out the food choices you'll want to make in order to promote weight loss and maintain a healthy weight, and I offer the science to back it up. Exercise is in here, too. However, I don't take up much space telling you what to eat and not eat and why you should exercise. And, though they are essential to personal success, it's not where I expect you to spend the majority of your effort, either.

Where you will be spending most of your time is examining the complex phenomenon known as human behavior and its unique relationship with food. Examining the way you as an individual think and feel about food and changing the ingrained habits that drive your food decisions is the soul of Brain-Powered Weight Loss. You won't be hearing much about theory; this is all about practice—a totally new and different approach to losing weight and making it stick. Not only is it designed to change your relationship with food, but the new practices you will develop are transferrable to other aspects of life as well. Try the exercises, techniques, and worksheets. I believe you will be more than pleasantly surprised at the change they inspire. You might find them transforming.

I recognize that humans are complex individuals with different needs and different emotions. You may find some practices I recommend irrelevant to your life, but you'll find many more that will strike a chord and become life-changing. If this book helps you make one meaningful change that impacts your life and reverses your personal battle with your weight, then I feel I've done my job.

Eliza Kingsford

INTRODUCTION

Why Diets Fail ... Every. Single. Time. (And This Plan Doesn't)

I am a licensed psychotherapist specializing in weight management, food addiction, body image, and eating disorders. I am also the executive director of Wellspring Camps, a total immersion weight-loss program for children and young adults up to age 26 that has the distinction of having one of the highest success rates in the world of people who lose weight and—here's the clincher—*keep it off.* I spend every day in the trenches with people who struggle with their weight. I know what their diet demons are, and I know how to get rid of them. I am also a member of the RiverMend Health (corporate owner of Wellspring as well as several addiction centers) Scientific Advisory Board, a panel of the world's best minds in weight loss and addiction, and am aware of all the research on what works best and doesn't work at all.

Brain-Powered Weight Loss is the culmination of all this knowledge. It is a how-to interactive *work*book that will encourage you to approach weight loss in a refreshing new way using the most sophisticated tool in existence: your brain. It is not something you'll read once and put on a shelf. It's something you'll want to come back to time and time again. It is a tool of practice—and power.

It's no secret that there's an obesity epidemic in America. While the reasons are many and somewhat complex, here's a major one and it concerns me the most: We are an obesogenic society. As a society, we talk a good talk, but we don't walk the talk. There are hundreds of books touting healthy eating and the latest trends in foods that are better for us nutritionally, but as a population we continue to gain more weight. Although there is a perception among some that we are eating healthier, our actions say something different. Americans spend $50 billion a year on products advertised to help promote weight loss, yet an estimated 70 percent of American adults are overweight or obese, and the rate is projected to rise to 85 percent by 2030. Think, for a moment, what this is telling us: If you are at a healthy weight, you are in the minority! The statistics are even scarier for children. The rate of overweight and obesity among them is an unprecedented one in three, and it's only expected to get worse.

Fifty *billion* dollars? Clearly, we are *desperate* to lose weight, and I'm here to tell you that the reason it's not happening cannot be blamed on us as individuals. There are just too many forces working against us that are out of our control.

First, as you've undoubtedly noticed, our food industry in the past 60 years has changed dramatically. We've seen the emergence of packaged foods, frozen foods, ready-made foods, low-fat and fat-free foods, and 100-calorie-pack easy-to-grab foods. In order for these types of "convenience" foods to exist safely on our shelves, they have to be processed, engineered, and chemically enhanced in more ways than we care to know about. Like it once was with cigarettes, I believe that we didn't realize the impact these "convenience" foods would have on our bodies. But we are seeing it now through our surging obesity epidemic. Many of these so-called foods shouldn't even be called food because we can't recognize a single ingredient on their labels. As far as I'm concerned, they should carry a warning label, just like cigarettes now do!

For instance, take the low-fat, no-fat, "lite" trend that's been all the rage for the past few decades. When you take the fat out of a product, you have to replace it with something else to retain a favorable taste, and that replacement is almost always refined sugars and/or artificial chemicals. When natural food is manipulated to such a degree, it falls into the category of "highly processed," which has created another phenomenon: food addiction. That's right, science has confirmed we can get addicted to certain foods, something you'll hear more about as you read through this book.

Even many packaged foods advertised as healthy really aren't, because our bodies weren't built to identify these added chemicals as fuel, so we end up storing what we're eating as fat. They also spike our insulin level and contribute to inflammation, a marker for many chronic conditions. Check the labels on so-called fat-free cookies, crackers, and snacks and see how many ingredients you are able to identify. I bet you won't find many.

In addition, marketers are spending billions of dollars every year pushing unhealthy, unnecessarily fatty and processed foods in front of our faces. They'd probably push them down our throats if they could. This is not unintentional; they know exactly what they are doing. Magazines and newspapers are flooded with stories about how to get the "perfect" body, ways to exercise more, and tricks to lose weight. Yet, tucked between those pages and plastered all over television are advertisements promoting the most caloric, fat- and/or sugar-laden products you can find. When you think it can't get any worse—1,100-calorie fast-food burgers, 850-calorie "salads," 300-calorie candy bars disguised as "health food," for example—it does. Really, do we need a pepperoni and cheese deep-deep dish pizza wrapped in 3½ feet of bacon, or deep-fried pickles to go with our double cheeseburgers? I can't imagine anyone thinks we do, even the people who come up with these concoctions.

If you're thinking, "But I don't eat any of those things, and I'm still gaining weight," consider this: Sensationalized messaging only serves to nudge our perception of what's normal or healthy in the wrong direction. If bacon-wrapped deep-deep dish pizza is over the top, it only makes a sausage and pepperoni pizza seem normal. I mean, really? This in itself is a problem because the more we sensationalize the extreme, the more extreme normal becomes.

Another reason we have an obesity epidemic in this country and in other parts of the industrialized world is because our modern society so easily fosters the problem. Sure, the fact that we drive everywhere instead of walk, and spend hours a day inertly staring at computers and social media instead of being active is part of it. At least these are things we can work on changing. The bigger problem is something we as individuals can do little, if nothing, about: the unapologetic marketing messages that are continually trying to tempt us with mouthwatering-looking food filled with nutrient-deficient empty calories. And marketers are doing it around the clock. We exist in an environment that is working against us. Trying to eat healthy day in and day out, from one meal to the next, is like continually swimming upstream. It takes a lot of effort!

For example, portions in a lot of restaurants, particularly popular chains, have gotten way out of control, and the fact that most chains must post the nutritional counts of their dishes isn't having much of an impact. They just reinvent the definition of a portion size as "meant to share," even when it all arrives on a plate for one. It's a blatant invitation to overeat. These days when dining out, you can be sure of these three things at a lot of restaurants: Portion sizes are too big; salt, sugar, and fat are generously added to accentuate flavor; and the quality of food has been compromised to account for costs. Trust me,

I'm not doggin' on restaurants, as I'm a huge foodie. But I make it my business to pay attention to these three things when I eat out.

The food you get at fast-food establishments is loaded with additives, preservatives, and salt, and the reason the prices seem like a steal is because quality is being compromised. Go back up the food chain and you'll find cattle being raised on cheap feed or corn instead of grass, which gives them chronic inflammation and nutrient-depleted meat that is passed down to us.

HEALTHY OBSESSION: YOUR STRONGEST DEFENSE

I'm not saying that these industries are intentionally trying to make people fat, but they surely are not doing anything to stop it. It is hard to stay healthy in a society that has set us up to fail, but it is not impossible. What it takes is a type of resilience that I call Healthy Obsession, an *intentional* mind-set—hence, obsession—so positively charged that it can help shield us against all obstacles.

The necessity for a Healthy Obsession is a new phenomenon, born to counteract the obesogenic movement I just described. Three generations ago—before Ronald McDonald was "born," before mac and cheese came in a box, before the TV dinner was invented, before two (or more) cars in every driveway became the norm, and before we could answer the phone or change the channel without getting out of our chair—being overweight was the exception, not the rule. There was really no need to have a Healthy Obsession. Back then, living a healthy lifestyle came more naturally. People ate fresh, whole foods and kept the body in motion to get chores done and get from one place to another out of necessity. In the 1950s, only one out of 10 people were overweight. Look at us today.

I am not suggesting we need to give up the perks and cushy existence of the 21st century. That's not what having a Healthy Obsession is all about. Having a Healthy Obsession simply means striving every day to live a healthy lifestyle by adopting the habits that make us prefer natural whole foods, feeling the need to stay active throughout the day, and ignoring the marketing messages that try to get us to do otherwise. When you approach life with this attitude, weight loss happens and it sticks.

I am not overweight, but I can guarantee that I would be if I didn't possess a Healthy Obsession. It's in my genes, and it's in my general nature. I actively live with a Healthy Obsession to keep my mind and my body in a healthy space. I can't imagine living any other way. For me, living a healthy lifestyle is just automatic. Every morning I wake up with an intention for how I'm going to live my day, and I focus on the behaviors that are going to get me to that goal. I call this an obsession because it is on my mind *every single day*, and that includes weekends, holidays, when I'm traveling for business, when I'm stressed and busy, and even when I take a vacation. It's not a place of anxiety or stress for me, and it never makes me feel deprived. My Healthy Obsession is my comfort zone, and I want it to become yours, too. It's absolutely possible, because I've seen it happen to thousands of people right in my own workplace.

THE WELLSPRING ADVANTAGE

Most of the people who come to Wellspring have a lot of weight to lose, some 100 or more pounds, which puts them at the highest risk for gaining it back. Yet, during the last decade, more than 10,000 Wellspring grads have made the Wellspring method the gold standard of weight-loss success. Most of them have become Long-Term Weight Controllers—or, as they call themselves, LTWCs—a badge they wear with pride. A professional review of 22 weight-control studies published in the medical journal *Obesity Reviews* found that behavior-centered programs such as Wellspring produced a 191 percent greater reduction in weight loss at the programs' end than approaches that did not include behavior therapy. And at follow-up, behavior-centered programs showed a 130 percent greater reduction in continued weight loss.

Wellspring achieves its remarkable results by putting its clients on a habit-forming, lifestyle-changing program that encompasses eating healthy whole foods they love, engaging in daily activities they enjoy—*love and joy* being key—and cultivating consistent, healthy behaviors about and around food, which is imperative. Here's what makes Wellspring different: When its clients are not learning about healthy eating or exercising, they are immersed in behavior-changing therapy targeted to transform them from a person who is obsessed with eating to someone who thinks like a healthy person—someone not just striving, but actually *desiring*, to eat what is good for them. At Well-spring, attaining a Healthy Obsession is a goal so powerful that the phrase has become our mantra.

Finding *your* Healthy Obsession is what this book is all about. As you'll discover, losing weight and keeping it off have absolutely nothing to do with dieting. In fact, there is plenty of scientific evidence showing that going "on a diet" can backfire—quite often big-time. Healthy Obsession is a set of behaviors that will change your lifestyle from one that promotes overweight to one that avoids it. Ingrained behaviors may be hard to change, but they definitely *can be* changed. Thousands of graduates of Wellspring are the proof. Here's how I'm going to help you go about it.

THE NEW AGENTS OF CHANGE

The behavior therapy program used in this book is based on the same approaches we use at Wellspring, but is customized for overeaters of all ages to use on their own at home. It is nothing like the antiquated behavior modification programs that have been around for decades and have had little, if any, impact on our food psyche. I will get you in a new contented state of mind using two types of cutting-edge talk therapies: Cognitive Behavior Therapy (CBT) and Dialectical Behavior Therapy (DBT)-informed principles, the same as we do at Wellspring.

CBT is one of the most highly researched and effective forms of therapy in the world, and hundreds of studies have proven that it can train your brain to change the way you think about *anything.* I have customized it to address the destructive habits and mind-talk that lead to overeating. Emerging 21st century research, including studies conducted on the Wellspring program, shows that successful weight losers who practice CBT are much more likely to maintain their weight loss than people who follow a maintenance diet alone. Or, as one recent study noted, "Cognitive behavior therapy improves adherence and decreases desertion of a weight loss program"—the exact goal of this book.

The DBT-informed principles I use in this book focus on the theory of the opposing ideas of change *and* acceptance. For example, DBT teaches us how to accept ourselves as we are—"Being overweight does not mean I am flawed"—while working to change—"Losing weight will help improve my confidence and self-esteem." It also helps us find and engage in behaviors that are least harmful to us on the way to achieving our ultimate goals.

CBT and DBT principles work because science has demonstrated that the brain has the ability to physically change at any age as a result of continually practicing something new—like changing your behavior around food. At one time, scientists thought the brain was wired at birth, but they now know this is not the case. Brain scans show the brain is malleable throughout life, what scientists call neuroplasticity. Through continual mental practice, we can physically change the brain's neuronal patterns and reprogram our mind in the way we think about food. Healthy whole foods cannot only become as desirable as chocolate cheesecake, they can become our preferred choice, the proverbial no-brainer.

CBT and DBT principles are the ideal mesh for success because both therapies highlight important links between what you think, how you feel, and what you do as a consequence. They then focus on replacing unsuccessful patterns of thinking and behavior with new, more useful ones. The techniques used in the pages that follow were all custom designed to specifically address the issues associated with food addiction and diet regression. It's not just how we feel that triggers us to eat; it's what we *think* that creates the feelings that result in overeating. Change your thinking pattern and you change the consequences.

But enough of the psychobabble. As you go through the exercises in this book, rest assured that everything you will be learning is all based on these two well-documented and studied therapeutic approaches that *work*.

HOW TO USE THIS BOOK

There are dozens, if not more, diet books and programs in the marketplace that tell you what you should eat to lose weight and how you should exercise to burn calories. But that's not this book. Why? Because you've probably been on your share of diets and already know what you *should* eat and that you *should* exercise—but still you're not doing it. You try, probably really hard, but you just can't make it stick. So, enough! That's not where I intend to take you. Instead, I'm going to take you on a weight-loss journey to where you've never been before, one that's focused on *how* to adopt the behaviors that will be your path to your ultimate goal: living a new healthy lifestyle. Here's how it works:

Your journey begins in **Step 1: Cultivate a Weight Loss State of Mind**, where you'll find out what Healthy Obsession is all about and make a pledge to pursue it by designing what I call a Decision Balance Sheet, setting up a self-accountability system, and writing letters of intention to yourself.

You'll truly find yourself in a different, perhaps even uncomfortable, place in **Step 2: Face Your Biological Truth** when you meet your personal weight-loss enemy—your biology. The body of most every person with a weight issue strongly resists maintaining a healthy weight. It's why other diets don't work. Understanding and remembering this will be your key driver of change.

Getting mentally involved in creating change starts in **Step 3: Identify Your Thinking Errors and Food Triggers** when you learn how to spot what's been derailing your good intentions. This is where you begin the process of reprogramming your mind to make decisions with intention.

Learning how to accept *and* change your situation at the same time comes into play in **Step 4: Find Your Wise Mind through Mindfulness.** It's all about awareness and learning to focus on the here and now—what I call living in your Wise Mind—rather than being on autopilot and reacting with your emotions. Mindfulness is an important practice because mindless eating is a key cause of overweight.

You'll learn the key processes to reversing your thinking errors and arresting your food triggers in **Step 5: Learn Your Dealing Skills—Then Use Them.** Mastering these skills is the big step forward to training your brain to adopt new behaviors. It's also the place you'll come back to time and again when you feel your behavior needs a little fine-tuning.

Step 6: Adopt a New Lifestyle of Healthy Eating introduces you to my healthy whole foods plan. It is not a diet per se—eat this today, never eat that *ever*. Rather it is a set of 10 nutrition principles that will teach you and empower you to eat the kind of foods aimed at defeating food addiction, producing weight loss, and maintaining long-term weight control. It's the core of what Healthy Obsession is all about.

You know you should exercise, but you don't. The reason? You haven't found the motivation. **Step 7: Make Room for More Movement in Your Life** doesn't so much tell you what to do (yes, there are a few "musts"), but offers the tools to find the motivation and, most importantly, make it happen.

Setting a big-picture goal to lose 30 pounds (or whatever) is going about it the wrong way. **Step 8: Set SMART Goals and Plans** shows that you will increase your ability to succeed and your sense of self-efficacy by learning to set and achieve goals that are specific, measurable, attainable, realistic, and timely—SMART—*every single day.*

Temptation is everywhere and nobody is immune. So you give in—and it's harmless, as long as you follow **Step 9: Prevent a Lapse from Becoming a Relapse.** Here's where you'll learn techniques to prevent and halt overeating, such as the art of harm reduction, a skill you'll use frequently to keep your emotional composure and prevent extremes—such as an all-out binge—from warping your judgment to get back on track.

Diet demons are everywhere! **Step 10: Outsmart High-Risk Situations** gives you the skills to take assertive actions and practice the mental filters that thwart the food pushers, circumstances, and situations that frequently come between you and your goals. It also offers alternatives to overcome 20 of the most common high-risk situations.

Step 11: Cross the Bridge to Healthy Obsession is the way you want to see yourself for the rest of your life. To cement your commitment to being an LTWC, you will make a contract with yourself to remain vigilant and on the path of continued success.

I recommend that you first read through the book to get the big picture of how that running tape in your brain operates and how this program works. Without a doubt, you will relate to most of what you read. Then go back to Steps 1 and 2 and start getting mentally involved. It is important for you to do the activities in these two steps before moving on. Reread the steps, and all steps, if necessary. It is best if you engage in all the activities in the next nine steps, but it is not necessary for you to do them in any particular order. Let your own needs be your guide.

For example, you may find that you are particularly vulnerable to regressing in your weight-loss efforts and beating yourself up over it, so you might want to concentrate on the skills found in Step 9. Perhaps you see that you aren't particularly good at setting goals, so you might want to take a first crack at Step 8. While you're actively participating in the book, you'll want to simultaneously start implementing the nutrition principles outlined in Step 6 and take the measures recommended in Step 7 to step up your activity level.

Practice and repeat until it sticks. *Stick-to-itiveness* is what will make weight loss happen this time and will make maintaining it a reality. You'll realize the revealingly positive impact it will have on your weight, self-compassion, body image, food obsession, and health.

GET READY, GET SET ... THINK

This book is the weight-loss friend on which you can depend. As you move forward in your Healthy Obsession, you'll want to come back and interact with it from time to time, especially during the ups and downs of life when your mind wants to go back to its default setting—your old way of thinking.

I have left space on the interactive parts of this book for you to write your responses. You also can find downloadable copies of all the exercises found in this book on my Web site, www.elizakingsford.com. This will help you to better keep track of your changing thought processes as you go through the program.

No matter how many times you've been "on a diet" or how many times you've been through the yo-yo cycle of gain-lose-regain, I have refreshing news for you. If you have this book in your hands, it means you still possess the drive to become a healthier you—and that's what's going to make the difference this time. You have the ability to power yourself into the self-image you see in your mind's eye. You are going to lose weight for good this time because you're finally going to get what it really takes. You are going to become an LTWC and realize what it's like to have Healthy Obsession.

Remember: Losing weight and keeping it off permanently is less about the stomach and more about the brain. So get out of the mind-set of "I'm on a diet" and into the thought processes that will launch you into a new lifestyle of healthy eating. Once you reach the mind-set of Healthy Obsession, it will never let you down.

Cultivate a Weight Loss State of Mind

I *hate* the word *dieting*. The reason is quite easy to explain. Dieting doesn't work. Period. Forget about it.

"But, but, but," you're thinking, "I've been on a *lot* of diets that worked like a charm." Twenty, 30, even 50 or more pounds lost. On some diets, it felt like the weight just melted away. You went from a size 16 to a 10, with barely a stop in between. And it felt like heaven.

Only look at you now. You're back to where you started from or, more likely, looking and feeling even heavier. And it feels like hell.

It's why I don't like the idea of dieting, and I bet you don't either.

The problem with going on "a diet" is that it implies there's a start and a finish—a life on hold as you miserably limit yourself with too little food and exert yourself with too much exercise until you just can't take it anymore. And that's the whole problem. "Dieting" is unrealistic because *it is not sustainable.*

Sure, there are lots of diets that work. Some, in fact, can produce amazing results. They deliver on the big promise. "Lose 10 pounds in 2 weeks!" "Drop three sizes in 3 weeks!" "Melt it off without moving a muscle!" But they all fail miserably when it comes to *true* success: The ability to sustain the diet and maintain the weight loss just aren't there. That's because the typical weight-loss diet works the same way as the typical pharmaceutical drug. It masks the symptoms but does not correct the cause. Go off the medication—or, in terms of weight loss, the "diet"—and the "disease" comes back. The rising world-wide obesity epidemic in both adults and children is proof of that!

That's what makes Brain-Powered Weight Loss so powerful. Unlike the hundreds of diets out there, this program does more than just treat the symptoms (overweight and obesity). It addresses a major cause—our problematic habits and behaviors around food and our mostly sedentary existence—and

1

puts the chronic diseases of overweight and obesity in remission. Here's the twist: The secret to losing weight and keeping it off is not so much about what we put in our stomachs; it's more about what we put in our brains, which brings me to Brain-Powered Pointer No. 1:

> Losing weight and making it stick
> starts with changing from a diet mentality
> to a behavior mentality.

When you change to a behavior mentality, you'll change your relationship with food. That's what getting in a weight loss state of mind—and its eventual success—is all about. It means forgetting about ever "going on a diet" again and following the path that will create for you a new style of *living and thriving*. How's that for incentive!

Why We Need a Healthy "Obsession"

The idea of being "obsessed" about health might sound like overkill, and it is. It's intended to be that way because that's what it takes these days to override the overwhelming outside influences working against a healthy quest.

When I first started counseling people struggling with weight loss and obesity more than 10 years ago, I made it my mission to educate myself about what is contributing to our obesity epidemic and why it is such a struggle for so many people to lose weight. I can say, with utmost certainty, that our current obesogenic environment—our 24/7 access to not just too much food but also too much unhealthy food and the marketing messages that promote them, as well as sedentary jobs and lifestyles—has made it nearly impossible to maintain a healthy weight and way of life without possessing an obsessive focus on the behaviors that get you there. If we were bombarded with marketing messages touting nutrient-dense whole foods the way we are with junk and other unhealthy foods, and if we were incentivized to move more the way our ancestors did, perhaps a Healthy Obsession might not be necessary. Unfortunately, I don't see that happening any time soon.

FROM A MIND-FOOD STRUGGLE . . .

Most of us struggle with weight loss because of our mental chatter. Our thoughts—our mind-set—drive our emotions, and our emotions drive our behaviors. Our mind-set dictates our eating choices and our urge to overeat, especially when we aren't even hungry. It's what makes us think, "To hell with it, I'll start the diet again tomorrow," when we stray even slightly from our weight-loss regimen. It's what keeps us out of the gym on "bad eating days," when we really should be motivated more than ever to go there. It's what makes us turn 6 weeks of dutiful dieting into an all-out binge on a lonely Saturday night. It's what makes us herald the holidays as the season to overindulge so we can start getting strict with ourselves all over again in January, just like we did last year and the year before that. And it's our mind-set that causes anywhere from 50 to 80 percent of us (depending on which statistics you want to believe) to give up the New Year's resolution and vacate the gym come February.

These types of behaviors occur because most people think of losing weight as being black or white—"I'm on a diet" or "I went off my diet"—flawed judgment that pushes our emotional pressure points of vulnerability and leads to defeat. The 11-step behavior-adjusting and lifestyle-changing program you are now embarking on has the power to break these barriers, and it starts with preparing yourself for change by getting in a weight loss state of mind. It means more than just telling yourself that this time is going to be different. It means *believing* it and *living* it. This time is not about going on a diet, it's about choosing *behaviors* that will change your relationship with food and lead you to desire a healthier lifestyle that includes eating healthy whole foods and getting more movement in your life. This time is not about taking a journey of abstinence; it's about taking a journey of substance.

This 11-step journey will take you through a series of scientifically based mind-strengthening exercises designed to move you from a subconscious state of complacent self-defeat to a fortified will to achieve and maintain a healthy lifestyle, what I call Healthy Obsession. When you build one new strength, it leads to another, then another. You will be able to achieve weight loss and become a Long-Term Weight Controller (LTWC).

. . . TO WEIGHT CONTROL NIRVANA

But what exactly *is* Healthy Obsession?

Healthy Obsession is not a fad and has nothing to do with loving only "health foods" or going to extremes in the name of health. It is more than having the stamina to sacrifice your desire for french fries and choose a sweet potato instead, or knowing that tuna tartare is a better appetizer choice than fried calamari. It is a permanent state of mind that gives you the desire to be healthy, eat healthy, and lead a healthy lifestyle. It's about possessing a set of positive behaviors you've built over time that have completely changed your thought patterns about food and exercise. When you have Healthy Obsession, you don't pass on the french fries with mouthwatering regret; you pass on them because you know that having a sweet potato will serve you better. It's about obtaining and possessing a state of mind as powerful as an elite athlete's drive and determination to set world records.

Healthy Obsession is not fantasy. It is so real and so relevant it is even scientifically acknowledged. According to a study on Healthy Obsession published in the medical journal *Childhood Obesity*, "Highly successful weight controllers nurture strong healthy obsessions" and "develop a preoccupation with the planning and execution of targeted behaviors to reach their goal." These 11 steps will lead you to becoming one of them. Which brings me to Brain-Powered Pointer No. 2:

> Changing your behavior from a
> food obsession to a Healthy Obsession will
> make you a Long-Term Weight Controller.

When you have Healthy Obsession, your focus is always on what best serves you—the choices you make that will get you to lose weight and maintain it, and prevent it from coming back. It's not so much that you don't want french fries; you simply prefer a healthier option. When you possess it, the decision between a doughnut or an apple for a midmorning snack is automatic. The optimal choice happens because you possess the desire to make it happen. It's not that you will never eat french fries or potato chips again; once you change your food mind-set, you'll desire them less, not care for them as much as you once did, or possibly not even like them anymore. Study after study has shown that it works.

People who possess Healthy Obsession—and I am one of them—describe it as a positive mind force that automatically leads to making the better choices when opening up the refrigerator or looking at a menu, without the remorse of wishing "if only I could" about somebody else's selection. It drives the way they think when it comes to food choices, temptations, and events that invoke the urge to overeat.

By repeatedly practicing the mental exercises in this book that create new behaviors, you can train your brain to desire the healthy choice because you fully grasp the consequences of what making an unhealthy decision will mean to your weight-loss goal, your ability to become an LTWC, and your overall health. Just as it is for me and the people you will hear from in this book (among others), Healthy Obsession can become part of who you are and the reason you will continue to achieve.

Dieting and Its Rebound Effect

Dieting isn't good for you. Not only do most diets eventually fail for most people, but research tells us that dieting has a rebound effect—you fail, beat yourself up over it, regain, and then put yourself through the whole cycle again. It looks like this:

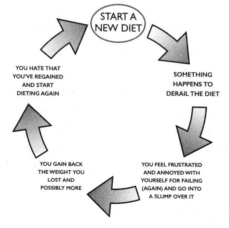

START A NEW DIET

SOMETHING HAPPENS TO DERAIL THE DIET

YOU FEEL FRUSTRATED AND ANNOYED WITH YOURSELF FOR FAILING (AGAIN) AND GO INTO A SLUMP OVER IT

YOU GAIN BACK THE WEIGHT YOU LOST AND POSSIBLY MORE

YOU HATE THAT YOU'VE REGAINED AND START DIETING AGAIN

How many times over the years have you gone through this cycle? It's what is popularly known as yo-yo dieting. Cultivating a weight loss state of mind is about making a commitment to change your behavior around food rather than making the commitment to diet.

GETTING FROM NEGATIVE TO POSITIVE

Yes, you *can* mentally motivate yourself to eat well, exercise and love it, and develop a passion for living an active and healthy lifestyle. Cultivating a weight loss state of mind begins with throwing out the concept of "diet" and instead making a commitment to change to a new lifestyle of healthier eating and healthier living. The following three exercises are designed to get you and keep you in a weight loss state of mind. You can complete these exercises in the spaces provided or download them from my Web site, www.elizakingsford .com. Look for them under these names: "Decision Balance Sheet," "Meta-Monitoring Diary," and "Letter to Self."

Design a Decision Balance Sheet

There are positives and negatives to every decision we make. Even something as glorious-sounding as a trip to Hawaii has some cons, such as a long flight, the high cost of staying at a resort, and the temptation to eat all that wonderful food. On the plus side, you get to spend a week or two relaxing, dancing the hula, and soaking up the warmth in paradise. Or let's take the decision to go to graduate school. You know that classes and studying will eat up most, if not all, of your free time. It's going to be costly, and it might feel like you're sacrificing a few years of your life. Now weigh that against the pros—an opportunity to get a better job in the field of your choice and the potential to excel and succeed. Worth the hassle? Only you can judge.

You may think that there are no negatives about losing weight—"OMG, I just fit into a size 6!"—but the reality is there will be some, if not many, challenges to making it happen. I'd like you to think about the pros and cons of weight loss in terms of your own life and past experience. This is an important, thought-provoking exercise, so I'd like you to take an hour or so of quiet time to think about it before you start writing. Think about all the other times you went on a diet and what led to failure or short-lived success. Think about both the physical and emotional aspects that hampered your spirit. Also, think about it in terms of losing weight by making a lifestyle change, not by going on a diet.

The Decision Balance Sheet is an important tool because it will keep you mindful of the reasons you're taking this weight-loss journey and the obstacles that are most likely to get in your way. To illustrate how to go about it, I'm going to use my client, Barbara B., a realtor who was in her midthirties and nearly 40 pounds overweight at the time we met 4 years ago. This is how she weighed her weight-loss pros and cons, based on her past attempts.

Good Things about Losing Weight	Challenging Things about Losing Weight
1. Looking great in clothes.	1. My husband is overweight and has no interest in losing weight. He may not like it if I get thin.
2. Making a better impression on my clients.	2. I hate to exercise and can never find the time.
3. Feeling good about how I'll look when I'm out with clients.	3. Giving up my convenience foods and finding time to cook healthy.
4. Not having to hide behind baggy clothes.	4. I have a sweet tooth.
5. Having more confidence in myself.	5. Monitoring my food choices and habits during the holidays and when I go on vacation.

Prior to doing this exercise, Barbara had never given much thought to her weight-loss challenges. She always thought of the good things and didn't even give much thought to what went wrong when her weight-loss effort failed. "Something always happened, usually some event where I totally blew my diet, and then I'd just lose interest," she told me. "Making this list really pulled everything in focus for me. I was able to anticipate and plan for the challenges ahead, and that made all the difference. I was able to overcome them." For example, when her husband mumbled something about "being on a diet," she would retort: "I'm not on a diet, I'm changing my lifestyle. I'd love if you'd join me." And, guess what, eventually he did! "He may not be the picture of Healthy Obsession, but he is more mindful about what and how he eats," said Barbara, "and he's starting to trim down."

She didn't lose 40 pounds, but she got close enough to experience her list of good things about losing weight, and she's satisfied with where she's at. "I'm selling more houses, and I swear it has a lot to do with the impression I make on my clients. I know that's because I'm so much more confident in myself now, and the people around me are picking up on that. I feel so much better about my appearance, and I think I carry myself differently now."

Now it's time for you to think about weight loss in terms of good things and the challenges. Do this first before all other exercises. Just as it did with Barbara, you'll see that it makes a difference. Keep this list in a prominent place where you can see it and read it often.

Affirm Yourself to Change

Affirmations are a type of practice in the power of positive thinking. The practice is based on the belief that you can restore self-confidence, foster a positive mental attitude, affirm a sense of self-worth, relieve stress, and curb negative outcomes by composing simple but carefully thought-out statements of self-empowerment that you consistently repeat aloud or to yourself. There is also evidence that affirming helps promote weight loss.

One small study, reported a few years back in the journal *Psychological Science*, divided women who described themselves as being dissatisfied with their weight into two groups: Those who affirmed and wrote about the values most important to them, and those who did no affirmations. After 2½ months, the research found that the woman who affirmed their values weighed less, had lower BMIs (a scientific measure of overweight), and smaller waistlines. Another study using brain scans demonstrated how affirmations possibly work: People who recited affirmations showed increased activity in the valuation system of the brain. The valuation system influences the choices we make.

I am among the legions of fans who strongly believe in the value of writing and repeatedly reciting affirmations. I have seen the difference it has made in hundreds of people on a weight-loss mission and in countless numbers of Long-Term Weight Controllers. Nevertheless, I have encountered people too numerous to mention who looked at me skeptically when I brought up writing affirmations as part of their mental reengineering program. "Just give it a try, even if you don't believe," I always tell them. "I

DECISION BALANCE SHEET

Good Things about Losing Weight	Challenging Things about Losing Weight
1.	1.
2.	2.
3.	3.
4.	4.
5.	5.

think you'll be surprised." And they always are. Now I say the same thing to you. You, too, will find that affirmations can restore enormous resilience in your self-confidence.

I will be encouraging you to write affirmations from time to time throughout this book. To be most effective, they should represent the four P's. They should be:

- **Personal**

- **Positive**

- **Pointed**

- In the **Present** tense

This affirmation exercise is very important to getting yourself out of a diet frame of mind and focused on making a lifestyle change. You can use this example or write one of your own:

I have the power to make changes; I have the power to change my lifestyle.

Every morning after you get up, perhaps while you are brushing your teeth, say this affirmation out loud and repeat it a total of three times. Or write your own affirmation here. Or, if you want to keep it private, write it in a journal or something similar. There is a document called "My Affirmations" on my Web site, www.elizakingsford.com, that you can download for writing all your affirmations.

Set Up A Self-Accountablity System

As you can see, Brain-Powered Weight Loss is an interactive program, so prepare to do a lot of writing. You can do much of the writing right here in this book, if you desire. But if you want to keep it personal, I suggest you get a three-ring binder and download the mental exercises as you do them from my Web site www.elizakingsford.com. You'll learn where to find them with each individual writing assignment. If you love journaling, then by all means get yourself a journal or start a My Weight-Loss Journey Journal file on your computer or tablet. In addition to the journaling required in the majority of exercises in this book, your self-accountability system also involves a food tracker and an exercise tracker, which I will tell you all about when you get to Steps 6 and 7.

Many people freeze at the idea of having to write about their private thoughts, because they can't think of the right words, don't know exactly what to say or how to say it, or fear they'll be judged. My approach avoids all these potential issues. I will be giving you plenty of guidance on what you need to say and how to say it. Most everyone who has tried these exercises finds them easy to do and personally enlightening. The whole idea is to help you discover where you might have a dysfunctional behavioral relationship with food and then use the proper tools to change it.

One practice you'll be doing is a quick daily check-in with yourself before you go to bed, in which you'll rate your progress and journal about your day's experience. It's called Meta Monitoring, and you'll be rating yourself on a scale of 1 to 100 or, if you'd rather, 1 to 10.

For example, one day you might give yourself a 98, or 9.8 and write, "A great day. Got lots of praise for my project at work. Stuck to my goals and my food plan to a tee and walked 5 miles. I felt invigorated." Perhaps the next day is not as good and you give yourself a 75, or 7.5 and write, "Stayed on plan but it was really a struggle; missed one of my goals (going to the gym), but I balanced it by walking 4 miles. Feeling bad because I had a fight with my mom and hung up on her." Two months down the road, you might hit a day that you measure as a 45 or 4.5 in which you record, "A near disaster. Found myself in a lot of cognitive distortions at the wedding, and I ate a lot of things that are off plan. On the positive side, I danced a lot and had fun."

The whole idea of this exercise is to check in and ask yourself, "How did I do today? How well am I measuring up to my goals? How am I doing with my behaviors around food and exercise? How are things going at work, in my personal life?" It's your opportunity to stand outside yourself and observe what you are doing and how well you are doing in relation to the goals you've created for yourself. If you're like most people, your Meta Monitoring will be a series of ups and downs. It's to be expected. As time goes on, you'll be able to see a link between your adherence to your goals and your behaviors and triggers. You'll be able to see the messages you are telling yourself and how they are driving your eating behaviors.

So, let's set this system up right now. Go to my Web site and download the exercise called "Meta Monitoring." Or design the exercise yourself in your journal or on the computer. It should look something like this:

META-MONITORING DIARY

Date:
Score:
Thoughts and observations:

Write Letters to Yourself

What does the mental snapshot of yourself look like? The way you look today, the way you used to look, or the way you wish you looked? What do you see and think when you look in the mirror? What do you envision your life to be when you lay your head down on the pillow at night? How do you look and feel in your daydreams? How does any of it or all of it compare to your life right now?

Most people believe that losing weight will make their life richer and more fulfilling in some personal way. They can even envision what their life will be like—walking the beach tan and thin in a bikini, standing straight and slender while giving a speech, getting involved in an exciting new relationship or reigniting a current one, becoming the salesperson of the year, or having the confidence to leave a circumstance that going's nowhere and move in another direction.

Having wishes and dreams and hopes of what life could be like "if only I could lose all this weight" is a fine aspiration; however, losing weight in and of itself is not going to make them come true. Feelings of empowerment, courage, self-confidence, and self-esteem only come with love and acceptance of yourself exactly as you are. They will only happen if you start *believing* in yourself right now. While losing a significant amount of weight can help you feel more self-confident, realize that the confidence comes from achieving a goal. And you have to believe in yourself in order to believe you have the ability to meet that goal.

You can start believing in yourself *now* and start cementing your resolve by committing to it on paper. The way you're going to do it is by composing two letters to yourself: the self you are now, and the self you want to become.

I know, you're probably cringing and saying to yourself, "I'm not doing this. It's not me. I don't know how to think about myself in these terms." Or "I don't want to write this stuff down. It's just too personal." I hear that a lot. I encourage you to do it, though, because this is the way you want to be thinking about yourself. It will get your vulnerabilities out in the open, offer you a purpose for taking this journey, and help strengthen your resolve when the going gets tough. Overweight and obesity in particular evolve for a reason, and it often goes much deeper than just giving in to the desire to overeat.

Your Letter to Self Now should address and answer this: What is it like to be you right now? Dig as deep into yourself as you can get. Be honest, blunt, and as raw as you can get. Think in terms of how your weight is affecting every aspect of your life, such as your self-esteem, marriage, children, sex life, social interactions, work habits, personal appearance, and physical and mental health. Your Letter to Future Self should express this: How do you envision your life will change after weight loss? Examine every aspect of it.

These letters are for your eyes only. There is no reason to share them if you don't want to. When you finish, tuck them away someplace where you can pull them out at a moment's notice when obstacles present themselves. And trust me, they will.

To help you out in this mission, here are sample letters written by a client I'll call Paul. He came to see me when he was 38 years old and 70 pounds overweight. He seemed so sad over where he was in his life, it made me sad. He gave me permission to use these letters as long as I changed his name and he could not be identified by the information, which is the same case for all the people you'll meet in this book.

Dear Self Now,

I've gotten so overweight I am worried I may not live long enough to see my children grow into adults and have families of their own. My last medical checkup was a disaster—high cholesterol, high blood pressure, and I'm on the verge of getting diabetes. And I'm only 38. Yikes! I know my wife worries about me, but I am also worried she could leave me. She rarely even gives me a kiss anymore and she's very distant. I know that if I keep on gaining weight I'll drive a wedge deeper between me and my family. The last thing I want is to become a burden to them.

Dear Future Self,

Beth and I are going on a second honeymoon. She's fallen in love with me again! Can't wait to show off my new physique on the beach after all the weight training I've been doing. My old vigor and my fun-loving spirit have returned. I no longer need blood pressure medicine, my cholesterol is normal, and so is my blood sugar. Yay! I now have the stamina and financial resources to take over the tire company when my boss retires in the next few years.

Sometime in the next few days, find a quiet place and contemplate your own life and where you want this journey to take you. Then start writing.

Now before moving on to Step 2, I want to address a question that every single person who is trying to lose weight asks me: How often should I weigh myself? Here's what I tell them.

WHAT TO EXPECT FROM THE SCALE

The scale can play a big role in your weight loss state of mind, as it can work for you or against you—or, more accurately, work *with* you or against you. Let me explain. One of the misguided ways many people approach a weight-loss plan is with unrealistic expectations. They expect to see the scale go down,

down, down with every weigh-in and feel an exaggerated sense of hopelessness when they see the scale go nowhere, and worse when they see it go up. But it will go up. *Expect it.*

Sustainable weight loss is never a straight downward line. It's more like the stock market, continually going up and down. It even has times of surprising highs and lows. A dramatic change in weight over a span of 24 hours—"Holy cow, I gained 2 pounds yesterday and I ran 2 miles"—does not mean that you gained 2 pounds of fat overnight.

Some people are so attached to the scale as a measure of accountability that they insist on weighing themselves every day. One client of mine, Stephanie R., is so dependent on the scale she purchased a high-end physician-style version with a digital readout, which allows her to track her gains and losses by the ounce. "It's my motivation," she says. "When I see it go up, even a little bit, I know I need to be extra vigilant that day." For Stephanie and people like her, a day without a weigh-in is a slippery slope that puts them at risk for reverting to the old habit of ignoring the scale, which can lead to engaging in former unhealthy eating habits. The scale helps keep Stephanie accountable to her new behaviors, and she likes it that way.

If that's you, then go for daily weigh-ins. However, you needn't take it to extremes. Weigh-ins are great if they don't stress you out, which brings me to Brain-Powered Pointer No. 3:

> Your relationship with the scale
> should be what works best for you.

For other people, the thought of stepping on a scale makes them too nervous and exasperated. They prefer weekly weigh-ins because they find days of ups and downs too deflating. Others don't want to step on a scale—ever. I know one woman, Jeanie P., who refused to use the scale and wanted to measure her progress by trying to get into an old pair of jeans. Her philosophy was, "I don't care what the scale says. I refuse to be beholden! I care how I feel and look in my clothes." This worked best for her because when she felt her jeans getting tight again, she knew it was time to tighten her behaviors a bit.

The scale is only a tool; it is not your judge. The way the body responds to its daily energy intake and output is too fickle to take the scale too seriously. I can't tell you how many times clients came to me with a lament like this: "I just don't understand what is wrong with me. I ate perfectly this week, didn't stray from my goals once. I exercised really hard. The scale didn't budge. Not a single bit. This whole thing just seems hopeless."

I cringe every time I hear this, because the scale is not a dependable gauge of your progress. Your weight is influenced by more than just the calories you eat and how much you exercise. There are numerous factors involved in the number that shows up on the scale, and they are largely out of your control. Fluid retention, stress, menstrual cycles, sleep quality, age, gender, your elimination system, and your emotional state are just a few of them. So my advice to you is what I tell everybody: If you are going to use the scale as a tool, use it to your advantage. If you find it motivating, go for it. If daily fluctuations and so-called plateaus—in which you can go for a week or even more without moving the needle—are too deflating, then find your motivation elsewhere. Turn to your non-scale victories, or what are called NSVs.

An NSV is any positive life experience that corresponds with your weight-loss efforts but does not show up on the scale. It can be your clothes feeling looser or moving to a smaller size; how your body moves (easier, faster, farther) when you exercise; a noticeable change in your energy level; a healthier change in the appearance of your skin, hair, and nails; or simply the ability to play on the floor with your grandkids without getting winded. In the end, it doesn't matter what the scale says day to day; what makes weight loss into a win is consistency over time. Stay in a weight loss state of mind and I promise, the scale will take you to where you want it to go.

THE STAGES OF WEIGHT LOSS

Losing weight is a journey mined with emotions that will, at times, challenge your weight loss state of mind. There are four stages of weight loss that people often go through on their way to Healthy Obsession. You may experience some of them. You may experience all of them. I believe that knowledge is power, and knowing they exist will help you recognize them for what they really are—just phases. They will pass! You will float in and out of them. Here are the four stages plus a fifth that is experienced by far fewer.

- **The Honeymoon** is your kickoff motivating phase. ("Wow! Six pounds in just 2 weeks!") It is so called because you want it to last forever. You're excited, maybe even exhilarated, and ready to make changes. Studies show that people who spend the most time in this stage produce better weight loss and weight control over time.

- **Frustration** starts to set in ("I didn't lose a thing for 2 weeks and then the scale went up!"). You begin to recognize that planning for weight-loss success can be time-consuming and, at times, even tedious. You start feeling the strain. This is when you'll need to use the skills you'll learn in this book to accept it and move forward.

- **Tentative Acceptance** happens when trying to lose weight starts to feel like a tentative reality: You see yourself getting there, but you realize it's going to take time and effort.

- A stage of **Ambivalence** usually enters months down the road when you start thinking, "Holy crap, this weight-management thing is going to be going on forever." Motivation starts to slip.

- Some people who see themselves losing a significant amount of weight will be confronted with a fifth stage of weight loss: **Fear of the Future.** This is when they realize they are presenting the world with a new persona. ("Will I still be me and will people like what they see?") This usually happens to people who start out obese and have a significant amount of weight to lose.

You may find yourself moving in and out of these stages many times. This is normal. Start expecting to fluctuate between moments of motivation and resolve, and moments of frustration and times where you'll consider giving up your new lifestyle. Crossing these hurdles means you'll be on course to Healthy Obsession, the winner's circle. You'll know you're there when you've conquered the goal of loving your new lifestyle—when you think the way healthy active people do.

The primary reason so many people go through some or all of these stages is because, when it comes to losing weight, the body isn't always in tune with your mind. Virtually all people who struggle with weight loss are up against a heavy resistance that few of us have ever even heard about before. That's where I'm taking you in Step 2.

MASTER OF WEIGHT LOSS: Terri C.

"Not Tomorrow, NOW!" Is Her Motto

I guess you could say I had a weight problem even as a young child, though I never really saw it myself. I was always the biggest among my friends and schoolmates in Bridling, England, but I was also very active and I loved swimming and playing soccer. However, I struggled with being fit—I guess because I was so big—and I sustained a lot of injuries that stopped me from playing. This is when my weight really started to spiral out of control. By the time I was 13, my mum was taking me from doctors to weight-loss specialists to dieticians. I joined gyms, dropped out, and rejoined others.

I remember joining this slimming club that my Nan took me to and hearing the consultant say, "Oh, yes, you do need to be coming here, don't you," as she looked over my shoulder at the scale. That really stung. It was my first and only visit there. For the next 5 years, I skipped in and out of different programs that I would now call "fad diets." I'd lose weight, then gain it back, plus more.

Things only got worse when I went to college. I was bullied and made fun of. Everyone called me "fat." I was devastated and became a recluse. I didn't want to go out anywhere. I totally lost confidence in myself and took out all my insecurity and boredom on the fridge. I topped out at 305. It's not that I didn't want to lose weight. I desperately did, but I couldn't find anything that would stick. I didn't even understand why I was so big. I didn't understand then, as I do now, that I was my own worst enemy. My mind was in a negative thinking pattern and I didn't know it. It affected my mood, which drove me to food. I was a classic emotional eater.

It was in 2011 when I went online and read about this weight-loss camp called Wellspring, but I wasn't sure how my parents could pay for it, or if they even would, considering all my past failures. I remember writing my mum a letter and putting it and the Wellspring brochure on her bed. They really wanted to help me and knew I needed the help. However, they told me, "We'll do this, but if it doesn't work and you get back into your old habits and start to gain again, you have to pay us back."

I never needed to!

As the time approached to go to the camp, I was so excited and I couldn't wait to get there. I ate like crazy, like it was my last supper. That's how bad my "food logic" was back then. However, when I showed up at the camp, I got so overwhelmed and frightened I wanted to go home. But I couldn't do that to my parents and, as it turned out, I'm glad I didn't because the experience has really changed by life. For the first time, I really began to understand why I was so overweight. My negative thinking would create emotions that drove me to food. The behavior classes I went through every day really flicked the switch for me. I worked closely with Eliza Kingsford to change my negative thoughts on life to a more positive way of thinking. She showed me how to build positive self-talk statements, which convinced me that losing weight was possible and gave me the confidence to give it a go. She taught me that an obsession does not have to be unhealthy and gave me all the tools to find my Healthy Obsession.

For the first time in my life, I learned about nutrition and portion size, and the effect different foods have on my body. I am now down 125 pounds and still counting. I'm my own "calorie queen," and I've been able to work out a personal nutrition plan that I enjoy and can live with. I wear a pedometer faithfully and go to the gym regularly.

I can't image ever falling back on my bad habits; I've learned too much. I am inspired by this quote from Deepak Chopra: "Every time you are tempted to react the same old way, ask yourself if you want to be a prisoner of the past or the pioneer of the future." I recite it every day. I tell myself every day and at every meal to stay on plan, and I don't allow myself to relapse—ever. When I get a craving, I talk to a friend or take a walk instead of going to the fridge. If I absolutely can't get rid of it—chocolate is my big thing—I can now take a small piece and be happy. Then I get back on plan with my motto: Not tomorrow, NOW! I can now go months without having a piece of chocolate when I used to eat it practically every day.

One of my most rewarding moments that will always stay with me is when I tried to carry my weight loss in a backpack at the gym. I could not stand up, let alone walk with it. I remember thinking, "How did I used to move?" That's motivation enough to never want to go back there!

Face Your Biological Truth

Most people can lose weight initially, if they commit to a program and stick with it. We've all seen it happen, and it may even have happened to you. But that's not what I call success. *True* success—that is, the ability to maintain a loss for 2 years and more—is fleeting. It comes to only an estimated 5 percent of people who go on diets, according to some statistics. Sadly, for all the rest, the weight rolls back on.

The reason so many people fail at weight loss comes down to two things: a society that constantly bombards us with oversized portions of unhealthy foods (I covered the issues behind this in the Introduction) and our own biology. Here's a biological fact few people know: The body of every single person who gains and then loses weight strongly resists the ability to stay thin. It's what I call Resistant Biology, and it's always working against you.

Simply put, Resistant Biology is an overabundance of fat cells in your body, the storage keepers of excess calories. We're all born with fat cells, millions of them. They are necessary for our survival because they release the excess calories they store when no other fuel is available to feed our bodies and brains. Back in the days when survival was a struggle, they conserved energy so we would not starve to death. If we didn't have fat cells, we wouldn't be here today!

Fat cells are physically capable of doing two things: They expand to their full potential, and then they multiply. Once they've multiplied, there is no going back. They can shrink to a more manageable size, *but they never go away.* Instead, they strive to survive. They like "feeling full," so they tend to want to cling to their calories. When we gain weight, we grow more fat cells. When we gain, lose, then gain again, we fill up the fat cells we added the last time we gained, and then we grow even more. The fat cells in the body of a yo-yo dieter can number in the *billions.* Science shows that once the body gets used to being overweight, it has a biological drive to return to its highest sustained lifetime body weight. Every time you add more fat cells, it becomes your new normal!

This explains why it can take you 6 months to lose 30 pounds and then see half of it roll back in as little as a month after going back to your old eating habits. If, for example, your weight peaked and settled in at 240 and you eventually get back down to 160, your new biology—programmed by your growing family of fat cells—wants to be 240 again. It's the classic cause of yo-yo dieting. You diet, lose weight, go back to eating like you did before, regain it all and possibly more, then go through the same cycle all over again as you accumulate more and more fat cells along the way.

If you have a history of struggling with your weight, more than likely you have Resistant Biology. It's why I hate the concept of dieting. Going on "a diet" implies there's a start and a finish. Life goes on hold while you unhappily work your way through the latest fad diet, all the while thinking, "This diet is the one that's going to work." Only it doesn't, and it makes your Resistant

ANATOMY OF A FAT CELL

The illustration, below left, is what fat cells look like in someone who has never been overweight: small in number and even in size. In the center, you can see what happens to fat cells when we take in more energy than we use: They expand and multiply in order to store fat. The illustration on the right shows what happens to fat cells after losing weight: They shrink but never reduce in number. This is because the body is designed to resist starvation by keeping its fat cells full, a throwback to the hunter-gatherer age when people had to forage and hunt for food and the timing of the next meal was always in question.

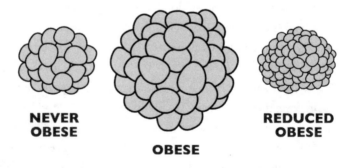

NEVER OBESE   OBESE   REDUCED OBESE

Affirm Your Resistant Biology

You can keep this indelibly in your mind by writing an affirmation that you should repeat to yourself every time you are making a food choice.
My Resistant Biology does not take a vacation;
always make the wise choice around food.

Biology jubilant. It knows it's only a matter of time before you go back to your old eating habits and start gaining all over again. And it's more than willing to accommodate by making room for more fat cells.

It's unfair, I know, but I am not dropping this reality on you just to bum you out. You *need* to know this. You need to never forget it. You need to acknowledge your Resistant Biology every single day. The reason? You can resist your Resistant Biology by working with it, not against it, which brings me to Brain-Powered Pointer No. 4:

> In order to lose weight and keep it off forever, you can't
> ever forget that Resistant Biology is part of who you are.

Know thy enemy. It's your prime motivator. People feel defeated after losing weight and feeling the pounds creeping back because they don't understand that their bodies are working against them. It's natural—it's *nature*. They get confused and frustrated. "How is this happening, and so fast? I worked so hard and my weight's coming back."

So, now you know. Just like people who have diabetes must be vigilant about managing their sugar and insulin levels, you need to be ever vigilant to the fact that your Resistant Biology is chronically trying to increase your body size. Like any chronic condition, Resistant Biology is a constant in your life. It doesn't care if you feel the need to eat because you're miserable or in a bad mood. It doesn't care if you're taking a vacation or celebrating a holiday. And it gives you no mercy because your spouse can eat practically all day long without gaining weight and you'd like to eat all day, too.

Acknowledging your Resistant Biology and understanding how it works is the pivotal first step you will make in readjusting your mental map. You can't make your Resistant Biology go away, but you can outsmart it by changing your food behavior. In fact, every exercise and practice you'll undertake in this book is designed to help you manage your Resistant Biology.

MEET THE RESISTANCE

Fat cells don't misbehave because there is a flaw in human engineering. They serve a significant purpose: to protect you from starvation, not abundance. Exposure to too much food is a modern-day phenomenon that the body does not acknowledge and probably never will (at least in our lifetime). Thousands and thousands of years ago, when cave people were foraging and hunting for

A Word about Your Health

You don't need me to be your reminder that the number one reason losing weight is beneficial is because of your health, so I'm only going to say it once: Overweight and especially obesity are strongly associated with chronic life-threatening diseases, mainly heart disease, diabetes, stroke, and certain forms of cancer.

Metabolic syndrome, also known as insulin resistance syndrome, is a cluster of five risk factors that heighten your risk of heart disease and diabetes. A leading cause: weighing too much and getting too little exercise. These are the factors associated with metabolic syndrome:

Overweight and obesity, especially too much weight around the middle, and what's known as being shaped like an apple. Men are more likely to be apples, although women tend to shift in this direction after menopause. The definition of having this risk factor for women is a waist measuring 35 inches and over. For men, it is a waist measuring 40 inches and larger.

High total cholesterol and, in particular, low HDL, known as the good cholesterol. The HDL cutoff for women is 50 mg/dL

and for men is 40 mg/dL. Total cholesterol should be under 200.

Triglycerides, another type of blood fat, that come in at 150 mg/dL or higher put you at risk.

High blood pressure. A consistent pressure of 130/85 or greater puts you in the risk category.

High blood sugar. A fasting high blood sugar of 110 or greater, as measured in a blood test, puts you at risk.

food, fat cells were their salvation. These were the well-studied hunter-gatherers you learned about in school who spent their days on the move, hunting for food without any assurance as to when the next meal would be. Animals were quite the rare catch, and fat cells were the assurance that a supper of fatty meat would be stored and preserved for future energy needs.

We may not much resemble the people of the caveman age, but our biological engines basically still operate the same. Our fat cells work on our behalf to store what we eat as fat and burn it later as fuel. They play a crucial role in sustaining life because they work as storage depots for nutrients, keeping them safe and on the ready to also serve as body fuel. Fat cells insulate our vital organs and keep us warm. They also feed our brain so it can function and think properly. We couldn't live without them.

While our biology hasn't changed much over time, our behaviors sure have. Nowadays, we don't even have to get up off the couch to shop for food; all we have to do is call or text in our order, and it will be delivered. As for keeping our bodies on the move, we are inclined to do so less and less. We don't even have to get up to answer the phone or change the TV channel. Our fat cells are still being triggered to store calories, but they are being triggered less and less to release and burn them! Every time you eat too much and move too little, your fat cells grow. Every time you gain weight, lose, and gain again, your body becomes more efficient and effective at maintaining higher-than-normal levels of fat—that's why it's called Resistant Biology.

Obesity is a complex issue, and scientists don't always agree on what contributes to the problem. However, evidence shows that there are a number of biochemical barriers that make losing weight and maintaining a healthy weight challenging. Fat cells are just one of them. Certain hormones are another, as well as our individual metabolism and our genes. It is in your best weight-management interest to know what these mechanisms are and how they act in your body, because what you're going to learn in this book will help make them work for you rather than against you.

Leptin

Leptin is a hormone secreted by your fat cells, which sends the signal to your brain that you're full—another reason why fat cells are useful. Only problem is, studies show that this appetite-suppressing hormone doesn't always work this way in people who are overweight and obese. It appears that when leptin levels get too high, they have a rebound affect: Their ability to turn off your hunger switch is nowhere to be found. Instead of signaling the brain that you've had enough to eat, the opposite is true. Rather than getting the message that you're satisfied, the brain believes you need to eat more and exerts a powerful force to do so, just as it would if you were starving. Scientists call this leptin resistance. Studies show that people who are obese have a tendency toward leptin resistance.

Ghrelin

Ghrelin is a hormone that works as an appetite stimulant, sending a signal to your brain that it's time to eat. It is manufactured in the stomach and tends to increase production when the stomach goes on low reserves. That makes sense—it's only doing its job! Problem is, studies show that as you lose weight, your stomach has a tendency to produce even more ghrelin, meaning this appetite-stimulating hormone gets more active. This is a major reason why sustaining weight loss is so difficult. Our ancient biological adaptations that were in place to keep us alive in the face of starvation thousands of years ago are now working against us. In the era of the hunter-gatherer, losing weight was a sign that malnourishment was kicking in. Ghrelin served as an antidote by turning on the appetite to encourage eating. The problem is, the hunter-gatherer's caloric demands are a thing of the past, yet our biochemistry is still reacting in the same old way.

Insulin

Another chemical involved in weight loss and weight gain is the energy-storage hormone known as insulin. It helps control the amount of sugar (glucose) in the blood and determines if it will be used as fuel (glycogen) or stored as fat. When you eat something that causes a rush of sugar into your bloodstream, your pancreas produces insulin to shuttle that sugar into storage. If your body detects it doesn't have enough insulin to move these calories, the pancreas will start producing more in order to guide the calories to their final destination.

Just as can happen with leptin, people who are overweight or obese can become insulin resistant. Their brains aren't getting the message that insulin has been released, so the pancreas puts out more. It's like trying to tune out a sound, only to have someone keep turning up the volume. When there is too much insulin streaming through your system, the body has only one place to store it—in fat cells. This is a major contributor to how the body builds excess fat.

The chief instigator of all this chaos is sugar, most specifically simple carbohydrates, such as refined flour and the added sugar found in processed and packaged foods. In contrast, when you eat nutrient-dense whole foods, insulin is slowly released into the bloodstream, just as nature intended. Whole foods are filled with nutrients, such as fiber, that your body uses to slow down the absorption of glucose into the bloodstream, therefore avoiding an insulin surge.

Cortisol

Cortisol is a key hormone involved in your body's response to stress. When we're faced with sudden stress—a deer jumps in our path as we're driving down the highway, for example—our appetite is suppressed and the digestive system shuts down in order for the body to release a cascade of hormones that allow us to react immediately. Cortisol and the hormone adrenalin flood into the bloodstream, mobilizing fat and carbohydrates out of storage so we have an immediate source of energy to counteract the stress.

The process of quickly supplying our body with energy was important during the days of the hunter-gatherer, who was often faced with sudden dangers—"Yikes, another saber-toothed tiger!"—and they needed plenty of extra energy to survive the ordeal. The effect, however, is short-lived. Though adrenaline quickly dissipates after the crisis is over, cortisol tends to stick around to turn the appetite back on, so we can replace all the energy we used up to fight the fearsome predator.

Only thing is, we aren't escaping saber-toothed tigers anymore. However, our bodies are still responding to stress—any type of stress—by increasing cortisol levels in the bloodstream. This is extremely troublesome to people with chronic stress.

Consistent high levels of cortisol have been found to inhibit weight loss and encourage fat deposits, especially in the belly. And it's not just happening during so-called fight-or-flight stress scenarios, such as slamming on the brakes to prevent hitting that deer. Even if you're cool as a cucumber, you could have a high stress *response*, meaning cortisol levels are high in your body most of the time. Studies have found that people who are overweight

Do the Genes Fit?

Are genetics working for or against you? It's easy to find out. All you need to do is look at your immediate family. Take a few minutes to answer these questions. Give them careful thought, then write down your answers here or in your journal, or download the "My Genetics" worksheet from my Web site, www.elizakingsford.com.

1. Are your parents and siblings at a healthy weight?

   _____

   _____

2. What about your grandparents, aunts, uncles, and cousins?

   _____

   _____

3. If not, who is not?

   _____

   _____

4. Have they gained, lost, and regained weight over time?

   _____

   _____

5. What struggles have you observed them having with their weight?

   _____

   _____

   _____

   _____

6. What similar patterns do you share?

   _____

   _____

and obese have higher than normal levels of circulating cortisol, or a high stress response.

Metabolism

Then, of course, there is your metabolism, which is the rate at which you burn food—what scientists call the thermic effect. Metabolism is part of the reason weight loss is such a difficult science. While we can say that it takes a 3,500-calorie deficit to burn 1 pound, we can't say for certain how long that will take. It depends on your metabolism.

When it comes to metabolism, everyone is different, something you undoubtedly know. Factors including gender, age, current weight, activity level, and stress all have an impact on your metabolism, which is why yours is different from everybody else's. It's why two people can weigh exactly the same, eat the exact same foods, and do the exact same type of exercise for the same precise amount of time, but not lose the same amount of weight. Frustrating, I know!

Now comes the part you're really not going to like. Every time you attempt to lose weight by restricting calories, your body turns down your metabolism. It's called adaptive thermogenesis, and it allows the body to survive on fewer and fewer calories over time—another throwback to your hunter-gatherer ancestors. This is why the process of starving yourself to lose weight doesn't work.

Adaptive thermogenesis is what allows someone to survive in the woods with only water for a few weeks or a lost soldier to get by on only a few nibbles of food a day until help arrives. It is also the reason why 14 winners of the television reality show *The Biggest Loser* eventually regained a significant amount of weight. According to the well-publicized 2016 study reported in the medical journal *Obesity*, their metabolisms simply did not recover from this slowdown.

Genetics

Last, but not least, are your genes. If you have a parent with Resistant Biology, chances are good you have inherited it. If both of your parents have Resistant Biology, then your chances are even higher. Studies show that children born to overweight parents are four times more likely to wind up with a weight problem than children born to parents who are naturally slim.

Studies of resemblances and differences among families offer indirect scientific evidence that overweight and obesity tend to run in families. Scientists have also identified variants in certain genes that may contribute to weight gain and the accumulation of fat cells. However, a genetic tendency toward being overweight does not make it a given. There is plenty of scientific evidence showing that overweight and obesity are, for the greater part, caused by "the interaction between behavior and biology." Scientists agree that genetics only plays a small role in the tendency to gain weight, about 30 percent. The other 70 percent is caused by an outside influence—your environment and the way you respond to it. Which brings me to Brain-Powered Pointer No. 5:

> A family tendency to be overweight need not be your destiny. Consistent awareness and behavior change can alter this trajectory.

Reflecting on the biological cards you've been dealt should serve as a permanent reminder that, yes, you are different than your friends who don't struggle with their weight. *You* must be forever vigilant about your behaviors. Changing your behaviors about and around food and exercise is how you're going to lose weight *this time* and overcome your Resistant Biology. Your behavior can even help change some of the biological actions that help make losing weight so difficult. For example, the kinds of food you eat can better control surges in insulin that promote fat storage. Avoiding processed foods, too much saturated fat, and foods high in added sugar can better control the hormones that control appetite. Getting more movement in your daily life and fueling your body with enough calories to keep you full of energy each day will help your metabolism run efficiently and effectively. You'll be working on techniques and tactics to counter all of the biological factors contributing to Resistant Biology throughout the rest of this book.

Changing behavior is all about consistency—consistency in the way you eat, in the way you move, and, most importantly as you are about to learn, in the way you *think*. In Step 3, we'll get on to the business of finding what these behaviors are and how they are affecting your eating habits.

META MENTORING WITH ELIZA

The Last 10 Pounds Are the Toughest to Lose

I consider Allyson, age 55, a star client. She came to me a little more than a year ago at 190 pounds—a lot considering her petite 5-foot-3 frame. She had crossed the BMI threshold from overweight to obese, and it raised the red flag. She was not just concerned about her appearance; she knew she was jeopardizing her health. She had been on countless diets since her college days, and each time she regained she got a little heavier—a classic example of Resistant Biology. Nevertheless, she lost 60 pounds in 10 months on my program. Now she sat in front of me exasperated. Not only had she not lost an ounce during the last 2 months, she felt herself gaining and couldn't figure out why. Here, we pick up in the middle of our conversation.

Allyson: I'm not getting it. I'm not doing anything differently than I've been doing since I got with the program. Heck, I could almost be the poster girl for Healthy Obsession, I'm that in love with my new healthy lifestyle.

Me: You got that right! I'm so proud of you, and I bet your family is, too.

Allyson: But I'm so frustrated because I can't lose 10 more pounds. Don't get mad—I know how you hate so-called diets—but I even went on a low-carb diet to see if that would work. It did, for a few pounds. Then when I got back into my healthy eating pattern, it came back—and I'm eating healthy! It seems like I'm stuck at 130, give or take a little.

Me: So, tell me what's wrong with weighing 130? Is that not an okay weight for you?

Allyson: Well, 120 is where I *want* to be. I liked how I looked at 120 and want to be there again. It's what I weighed when I went to college. And (she giggled) I got back down to it three times with dieting, even when I weighed 150.

Me: And you are older now. Metabolism slows down little by little as we age. You're 130, you tell me you think you look great, and you're happy and confident. Tell me, if you lose 10 more pounds, what will it bring to your life that you are not getting now? What will it change about you internally?

Allyson: I'd be a size 6. That's going to have to feel awesome! That's really all.

Me: Have you ever thought that maybe your body is just refusing to go that low? Maybe it's more comfortable at the weight you are now? Seems like the way you are exercising, moving, and eating now can support your 130 pounds. To move the needle, it looks like you'll need to decide if you want to be more rigid with your routine. Are you willing to do that?

Allyson: Well, that depends. What would I need to do?

Me: Right now, it seems you and your metabolism are copacetic. Losing those so-called last 10 pounds means you probably need to get really strict with yourself, and in a way that you may not be able to sustain for very long. For example, you'll probably have to put yourself on a regimen that involves things like closely monitoring and measuring the quality and quantity of macronutrients you take in and stepping up your exercise to a level and time commitment more so than what you're already doing. Things like conditioned athletes go through. I support you if those are your goals, but I want to make sure that's something you really want to do.

Allyson: No way I'm doing that! That's not *Healthy* Obsession to me. That's just obsessed! So you're saying it's impossible for me to lose the final 10?

Me: I am not saying it is impossible. I'm just saying it will probably take something more extreme to get you there. That's not natural for you. It seems like 130 is where your body naturally wants to be. You need to enjoy life. Following a healthy and active lifestyle has gotten you to a healthy weight, and it's a lifestyle you love and can stick with for the rest of your life. My hope for you is that you're able to be happy with how much you achieved. You're healthy and you are *not* overweight.

Allyson: You make a lot of good points. I'll just keep up with what I'm doing now and, who knows, maybe just wanting to lose another 10 will keep me motivated enough to at last keep me where I am.

Me: Good thinking!

There are many people like Allyson who have unrealistic expectations about how much they want to weigh. In fact, I'd say most people are the same way. It's a side effect of the too-thin images we are subjected to in the media. Don't worry so much about what the scale says. Look at what you see in the mirror and think about how you feel inside. If the last 10 pounds become impossible to lose, then let it go. Why make yourself miserable trying to get to a place you can't sustain. Just enjoy life instead.

Identify Your Thinking Errors and Food Triggers

Virtually everyone who struggles with a weight problem has diet demons that both consciously and subconsciously condition them to mindlessly overeat out of habit, stress, boredom, or other emotional triggers. We eat when we're worried: We nervously wait with one hand in a bag of chips while fretting, "OMG, my son is two hours late." We eat when we're stressed: A milkshake and fries accompany your lament of "I'll never get this report done by Friday." We eat when we're jubilant: "The deal went through! Let's go out to celebrate!" We eat when we're alone, just because we've got nothing better to do. And we eat when we're not even hungry, just because it's there: "My husband is eating, so I guess I'll have some, too."

Most people think that our emotions drive us to overindulge when, in fact, it is our thinking errors, or cognitive distortions, that do. Thoughts create our emotions: "My son's been in an accident" (worry), or "I'm going to get fired if I miss my deadline" (stress), or "Wow, a celebration—bring it on!" (good intentions get thrown to the wind). While most people would label this "emotional eating," it is really only part of the equation, which brings me to Brain-Powered Pointer No. 6:

> Thoughts create the emotions
> that drive us to overeat.

Change the way you think—"My son must be having too much fun at the party and lost track of time"—and you'll change the way you feel (calm, reassured) and the way you behave ("Time for bed, not chips") around food. In other words, steer with a wise mind instead of an emotional one.

As a psychotherapist specializing in weight loss and eating disorders, I see it all the time. People who struggle with a weight problem wrestle with thinking errors *constantly*, creating a relationship with food that is chronically problematic. For example, they think that "party" means "I deserve to overindulge," instead of "There will be plenty of food options at the party, so I will have no problem sticking to my goals." Or they think, "My husband's having ice cream, so why not me, too?" instead of "I'm not hungry, so I'm happy to just be with him while he's eating and talk."

These thinking errors are mental chatter that test our resolve to stick with our goals, lure us to make the wrong choices around food, and drive us to overeat. They create a life of their own by becoming our automatic thoughts, a veritable running tape in our head. These automatic thoughts dictate what we think about ourselves and create even greater distortions: "I've gained so much weight, I don't know how I'll ever lose it." And that becomes our *reality*. This is how people wind up in my office telling me, "I've gained 50 pounds, and I don't know how I got there."

When I explain thinking errors to many people, they don't quite get it at first: "Yeah, sure, I'm an emotional eater, but it's hard to turn off those emotions. I can't change the way I feel." True. You can't always change the way you feel, but you *can* teach yourself to become mindful of the thoughts that are creating the emotions that are causing unwanted and/or unhealthy habits and behaviors around food. Which brings me to Brain-Powered Pointer No. 7:

Change your thinking habits and
you'll change your eating habits.

THOUGHTS = EMOTIONS = BEHAVIOR

| COGNITIVE DISTORTIONS | = | EXAGGERATED EMOTIONS | = | OVEREATING |

COGNITIVE DISTORTIONS THAT LEAD TO UNWANTED EATING

Cognitive distortions are thoughts that create an inaccurate or exaggerated picture of reality in our minds. These types of thinking errors are like land mines charged with negativity that pepper your road to success. You never know when one is liable to explode and threaten your resolve. They are your biggest enemy because they diminish your self-image, self-worth, and mental stamina, thus hampering your determination to succeed and crippling your ability to make smart decisions. Cognitive distortions are often the cause of binges and the reason why people lapse and give up on a weight-loss plan.

Let's not let it happen to you. You can sweep those land mines and rewrite that running tape in your head so you can move forward more assuredly in your resolve for a new, healthier lifestyle—losing weight, feeling great, eating healthy, and getting on the move. For starters, let's get in touch with your thinking errors.

Here are 10 of the most common cognitive distortions that drive people to emotional eating. Most likely, you will be able to recognize yourself in a few or more of them. After reading each of the descriptions, check the box if it sounds like you, even if only a little bit. This is not meant to label you or demoralize you. Think of it as getting to know yourself a little better, possibly a lot better. As I said before, knowledge is power. Recognizing your own cognitive distortions is the first step you will take to power your own change and put that running tape in the shredder.

☐ 1. Black-and-White Thinking

Black-and-white thinking is probably the most common mistake I see among people who struggle with their weight. This mind-set creates an all-or-nothing cycle that pushes you toward failure as soon as one single thing goes wrong. "I hit the dessert tray—my diet's ruined!" Only it's not. Or "Damn, I ate my breakfast, then cleaned up my kids' plates, too. Forget my eating goals today!" Only you shouldn't. Or "I can't believe I bought chicken potpie. No point now in hitting the gym." But that's exactly what you should do. Or you step on the scale after a particularly austere week of sticking to your plan and discover you didn't lose an ounce—"That's it, I just can't lose any weight." But you can.

Black-and-white thinking is the mind-set of habitual dieters because they constantly see themselves as being either on a diet—restricting themselves from foods they love—or off the diet—eating "forbidden foods" with relish. One little misstep in your plan and it's ruination. It's back to the diet again tomorrow or, more likely, Monday or, what the heck, might as well wait until the end of summer when the kids are back in school. In the meantime, you indulge in the foods you crave because you know you'll miss them once the diet starts again.

Here's an example of black-and-white thinking. Let's say you caved and ate eggs Benedict and a side of biscuits when you went out for Sunday morning breakfast, even though your wiser mind was trying to convince you to eat a tomato and spinach omelet. When you think in black and white, you get angry and tell yourself you screwed up royally (again). You're deflated and beating yourself up. You see losing weight as an impossible task and may even abandon your plan right then and there. You end up wallowing away the rest of the day with your head in the refrigerator and worrying what you're going to see when you find the nerve to step on the scale.

People who live in black-and-white thinking fail to consider that there are *choices* between all or nothing. They have a difficult time getting back on track when deviation happens. They view their day as ruined instead of accepting that one decision was just one mistake and it's time to forget about it and move forward. When repeated over time, this kind of thinking creates a consistent barrier to success.

☐ 2. Overgeneralization

People with this mind-set see a single negative event as a never-ending pattern of defeat. It's the continuation of black-and-white thinking—a small misstep is turned into a blown-out-of-proportion event.

Let's return to that eggs Benedict breakfast as an example. "Not only did I order the wrong thing," you tell yourself, "but it happens every single time I go out for breakfast. What's wrong with me? Eating out is just not possible for me." You work yourself into such a tizzy over it, you start to question your self-worth: "I'll never get to where I want to be." You abandon your diet, thinking "What's the point?" until the next time you muster up the courage to start dieting again. Overgeneralization is a sure way to mentally talk yourself into failure.

☐ 3. Mental Filtering

You've lost 15 pounds and people are noticing. Your officemates are smothering you with compliments: "You look great!" "That new outfit really shows off your slimmer figure." Then you meet your mother for lunch, and she says, "You're looking tired. I thought you were working on losing weight and improving your health. How's that going?"

Forget the 20 compliments you heard that morning. All you can think about is the fact that your mother hasn't noticed what the people in your office are seeing. This is mental filtering. You pick out a single negative detail and dwell on it exclusively, to the point where it darkens your vision of reality, just like one drop of ink can discolor an entire beaker of water. It almost brings you to tears. You mope through lunch, all the while feeling self-conscious about the way you look. Your mind is not on the compliments or your lunch. It's on your weight, as you mindlessly eat your way through the bread basket.

Now think beyond mental filtering. In reality, perhaps your mother really did think you looked tired because she's worried that you're working too hard and not getting enough sleep. Maybe she didn't notice your weight loss because she's concerned about the strained look on your face. On the outside chance she ignored your improved figure out of a little jealousy, one left-out compliment should not negate the multitude of encouragement you heard all morning.

☐ 4. Disqualifying the Positive

Let's get back to those compliments from your co-workers. When you disqualify the positive, it means you're just not buying it. You think what your co-workers are telling you is not really true—they are just saying it to be nice. You think, "I'm still overweight and they know it."

Some people who are overweight have such a poor self-image that they can't see themselves in anything but the negative. If you struggle with your self-worth, this cognitive distortion could be a major contributor to your negative thinking pattern. You may have trouble viewing yourself in anything but a negative vision, so when someone does pay you a compliment, you immediately dismiss it as untrue. You discount positive experiences by telling yourself that they "don't count." You put yourself in a mind rut so deep you live in a negative shadow that is contradictory to your everyday experiences. When people feel bad about themselves, they make bad food choices.

☐ 5. Jumping to Conclusions

An attractively dressed woman stares at you at the grocery store, and you think, "Why is she looking at me that way? I must look horrible." That's jumping to a conclusion. This mind-set constantly interprets every experience as a negative without any evidence to support the conclusion. There are no facts, no fact-checking. You constantly make assumptions about yourself: "She's staring at me because she thinks I'm a slob," even if it's more likely that she's staring at you because she thinks she recognizes you from somewhere and can't put her finger on it.

People who jump to conclusions don't see themselves as others see them. They think others see them as they see themselves—and for those lacking confidence about their appearance, it is not in a flattering way.

When you're in this mind-set, you can jump to conclusions about *anything*. You play the mind reader, arbitrarily reading the negative in someone's actions without any evidence whatsoever—"Why is he staring at my double chin while he's talking to me?" when he's actually looking you in the eye. Worse yet, you tend to play fortune-teller, anticipating that something or an event will turn out badly, thereby helping to make it a foregone conclusion: "I just know I'm going to eat too much and all the wrong stuff at the party tonight."

☐ 6. Maximizing and Minimizing

You should be able to relish in your successes and accept your failures without judgment, but people in this mind-set have difficulty seeing it this way. Instead, they tend to magnify something they messed up: "I am certain the scale will be up at least 3 pounds and probably more tomorrow because I ate those stupid eggs Benedict." They also tend to minimize things that should please them: "I ran only 5 miles. I should be able to go farther by now." This kind of thinking destroys your confidence in achieving your goals.

People who are always maximizing or minimizing don't have the ability to give themselves credit for their accomplishments. Worse, they make excuses for what they've achieved: "The only reason I won is because there weren't many competitors." They have a tendency to take the blame when something goes wrong but don't give themselves credit for something that goes right. They overidentify with their perceived failures and attribute them to personal characteristics: "I overate again. I am such a failure." In this way of thinking, there is no way you can win.

☐ 7. Emotional Reasoning

You're the type of person who feels things very deeply and lets your feelings drive your actions, taking the attitude "I feel it, therefore it must be true." You *feel* you'll never lose weight, so you give up on yourself. You *feel* you'll never stick with an exercise program, so you skip the gym. You *feel* you'll eventually gain your weight back again, just like in the past. Your fears are a trajectory to your inevitable outcome. But the reality is that, with some practice and attention, it is just as possible to feel the opposite.

☐ 8. Can't, Shouldn't, and Mustn't Thinking

"I can't eat that. I shouldn't eat this. I mustn't go into that pastry shop." In other words, you're punishing yourself. You're living life in miserable deprivation. These are all negatively charged words that bring on guilt and snuff motivation. When you think in absolutes—"I can't ever have a milkshake again"—you are setting yourself up to fail. You are living in a sea of extremes and absolutes, a powerful mind-set that self-imposes limits and rules on yourself, which can take on a mind of their own. They do not serve you in any positive way. Not only do they make you feel like you're missing out, it becomes your reality.

Words like these require no action, so when you use them, you hit a dead end—you're stuck with no way out. In reality, you always have choices. Recognize this. You just have to consider the consequences. This is what motivation is all about. "I don't drink milkshakes" speaks your conviction, while "I can't drink a milkshake" is a reminder that you're missing out. One study found that people who speak in terms of "I don't" instead of "I can't" are perceived by others as having stronger convictions.

☐ 9. Labeling and Mislabeling

This takes overgeneralizing to the extreme. People do it all the time. Instead of recognizing the event—ordering the wrong breakfast food—as only an error, you turn it on yourself: "There I go again, ordering off plan. I'm such a loser. I can't get anything right." It's totally irrational. You are making assumptions about yourself without logical reasoning. However, when you label the *behavior* instead of yourself (or others), you externalize the event, which allows you to respond to a slipup with more reason: "That wasn't the best choice for me this morning, but I know I will make a better choice at lunch."

☐ 10. Personalizing

This kind of thinking occurs in all of us from time to time, but it happens a lot to people who always try to please others. You personalize when you attach an emotion to a result that was unintentional: "I should never have said that. It was so mean." Or you are quick to blame others, failing to look at what your role in things might be: "This project is such a mess. I never should have trusted my partner." Or you feel responsible for something that may have little to do with you: "I can tell from her mood that she's really angry with me," when, in reality, she's having a tough time at work.

Sadness, guilt, frustration, anger, anxiety, helplessness, and fear of disappointing or hurting others are among the many emotions we can bring on ourselves when we personalize the events of our lives. It's the perfect example of how thoughts lead to feelings and feelings lead to food.

GETTING IN TOUCH WITH YOUR THOUGHTS

Undoubtedly, there are at least a few of these descriptions that jumped out at you ("Yep, that's me to a tee!"); others maybe a little, but not so much. If this is the case, go back and mark them off anyway, if you haven't already.

Not to fret. There is no judgment. No one way of thinking is worse than another. There is no "uh-oh," even if you marked off all of them. Remember, knowledge is power. Recognizing that you have a tendency toward cognitive distortions marks your first step to bringing it into conscious awareness. Keeping it there takes practice.

The thought patterns you've identified are a synopsis of your internal dialogue, the tape that's been running in your head most, if not all, of your life. It is a reflection of your unconscious self—your core beliefs, shaped early in life, that have formed the relationship between the world and the way you perceive it. The graph on the next page shows you how it works.

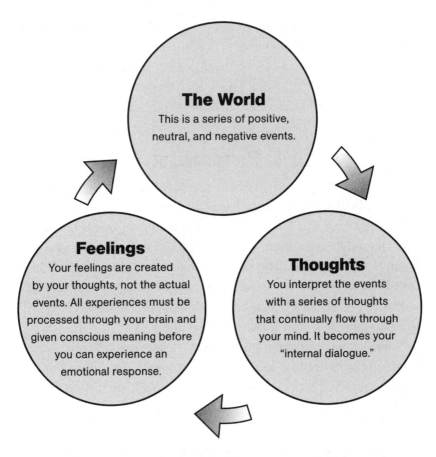

Now gather all the cognitive distortions you checked off and list them below or in your journal, or download the document called "Cognitive Distortions List" from my Web site, www.elizakingsford.com. If you're not sure and see yourself in kind of a gray area, then include it. If some part of it rings true, then it is something you're going to want to work on.

I relate to these cognitive distortions:

1. _____

2. _____

3. _____

4. _____

5. _____

Now you're set up for your first big assignment: training your brain to become acutely aware of your cognitive distortions. First thing tomorrow, start paying close attention to your thinking patterns. Are any cognitive distortions running through your head? Make a mental note of them and at the end of the day, mark them off in the space below. Or download the worksheet called "Cognitive Distortion Awareness" from my Web site and attach it to your journal or notebook. Do this every day for the next 4 weeks. By the end of the month, spotting these patterns should be automatic. If you're still not attuned to your running tape after 4 weeks, then carry on until you are.

This exercise is not meant to be done in isolation. Do it simultaneously with other exercises in the book until your awareness becomes automatic.

COGNITIVE DISTORTION AWARENESS

Week 1							
Cognitive Distortion	Sun	Mon	Tues	Wed	Thurs	Fri	Sat
1.							
2.							
3.							
4.							
5.							
Week 2							
Cognitive Distortion	Sun	Mon	Tues	Wed	Thurs	Fri	Sat
1.							
2.							
3.							
4.							
5.							

(continued)

COGNITIVE DISTORTION AWARENESS *(cont.)*

Week 3							
Cognitive Distortion	Sun	Mon	Tues	Wed	Thurs	Fri	Sat
1.							
2.							
3.							
4.							
5.							
Week 4							
Cognitive Distortion	Sun	Mon	Tues	Wed	Thurs	Fri	Sat
1.							
2.							
3.							
4.							
5.							

EMOTIONAL TRIGGERS TO BEHAVIORS

There are two factors that can cause undesired behaviors around food. One, obviously, is certain foods, which I will tell you about in Step 6. The other is our emotional triggers. Thinking errors and emotional triggers are intricately intertwined. A mood can change in a nanosecond—we've all experienced that! For example, let's say you're having a great time at your 10-year-old's birthday party until your ex walks in with his new squeeze, and suddenly you want to strangle somebody. Instead, you cut yourself another slice of cake. That makes your ex and his girlfriend (or each individually) an emotional trigger, an antecedent to unwanted behavior.

Emotional triggers are actually events, *neutral* situations that only take on a volatile life when we attach a thought to it. Your ex walks in the door with a new girlfriend and you think, "How dare he bring her into my home and in front of the entire family?" It makes you so angry you take it out on the birthday cake. If, however, you're glad he has a girlfriend because you have a new husband, you wouldn't have the negative thoughts and you wouldn't think

Meet Your Mood Evaluator

Food and mood do more than rhyme. Your mood directly impacts what kind of food and how much of it you want to eat. When we're in a good mood, we tend to make healthy choices, but when we're in a bad mood, we tend to make choices not in line with our goals. Research conducted jointly by Cornell University and the University of Delaware confirms that understanding why we make food choices when we're in a bad mood can help us make healthier choices. This exercise is designed to do just that. It will bring to the surface the automatic thoughts that lead to the mood that leads to your food choices.

Every time you're in a negative mood or feel yourself getting into one, come back to this mood evaluation exercise, which you can do here or download the worksheet by the same name from my Web site, www.elizakingsford.com.

Describe the situation that involves your current mood.

_____

_____

_____

_____

Describe your mood.

_____

_____

_____

_____

What were you thinking when you got in the mood?

_____

_____

_____

_____

twice about another piece of cake. Your ex bringing his new girlfriend to the party is actually a neutral event. It's the emotion that you attach to the event that makes it a trigger—or not.

We all have emotional triggers that drive us to overeat, or eat when we're not hungry, or eat when we feel the need to soothe. You can probably name a few off the top of your head right now. Thanksgiving, the holidays, vacation, and parties are obvious examples most of us share. That's right, triggers are not necessarily negative events. Oftentimes, the emotional link is something pleasant. For example, you might have a problem controlling your eating when you visit your Uncle John because you have a fond memory of him barbecuing ribs when you visited every Sunday as a kid. Or you can't stop yourself from veering toward your favorite funnel cake stand when you take the kids to the state fair because you subconsciously relate carnivals to indulging in special treats.

We all have events in our lives that we can directly associate with overindulging. In the space below, or in your journal, list all the events in your life that have the potential to cause you to overeat or not eat according to your plan. Or download the document "Triggers to Overeating" on my Web site, www.elizakingsford.com. Consult "Is It Hunger or Habit?" (at right) to help get you thinking:

1._____

2._____

3._____

4._____

5._____

6._____

7._____

8._____

9._____

10._____

Now you might expect me to tell you to just avoid them—problem solved. However, that is not the way it works. You should not avoid any of these occasions, as they are a part of the life that you enjoy. Rather, approach them in a way that successfully fits with your weight-management goals, which I will show you how to do in Step 10. For now, I want to help you identify triggers that are more insidious in nature, the ones that are so subtle you are not always aware they even exist.

I went through the experience recently with my client JoAnn B. She was down on herself because, two nights before, she had gone to an Italian restau-

---

Is It Hunger or Habit?

I know what is probably going through your head as you're reading this step: "I eat because I'm always hungry!" People tell me that all the time. But how do you define hunger? There is a difference between true hunger and the perception of hunger. True hunger starts in your brain when the hormone ghrelin tells your stomach, "You're empty. Time to eat!" It may even announce itself loudly through the sound of your stomach growling. It's a physical reaction to the need for calories for fuel. Beyond this, we choose food for other reasons.

Perceived hunger can always be traced back to a trigger, be it positive, negative, or neutral. These are common triggers that people typically associate with unintentional eating:

- Daily routines and habits, such as popping open a beer and reading e-mail after coming home from work, or putting sugar and cream in your morning coffee
- Special routines, such as holidays, family events (reunions, weddings, etc.), and vacations
- Boredom
- Seeing and smelling food
- Talking about food
- Being in the presence of food, like when you buy items not on your shopping list at the supermarket
- Fatigue
- Being around certain people
- Time of day, such as eating when giving your kids an after-school snack
- Surprising news, either good or bad
- Celebratory events
- Being around sugary or fatty foods
- Participating in events related to food, such as going to a ball game or the movies
- Procrastination
- Difficult emotions, such as anger, anxiety, grief, and sadness

rant with the best of intentions and found herself uncontrollably ordering the wrong things. She couldn't understand why she did it, as she was certain nothing had triggered her behavior. However, I will tell you what I told her: Something *always* triggers an unplanned eating event. I took her through a process of self-awareness called Chaining, and it went like this:

Me: What happened?

JoAnn: Well I'm not sure. I did everything right. I looked up the restaurant menu online and decided I was going to have pasta and shellfish in tomato sauce and a glass of white wine. I even roughly figured out the calorie count and knew I was in line with my goals. Everything was going fine, but for some reason I ignored my plan, asked for a menu, and ordered fettuccine Alfredo. And I don't even like it that much! My friend asked me if I wanted to share some fried calamari and I said, "Sure, why not?" even though I knew why not. I also ordered a big martini instead of the wine.

Me: Let's slow this down a bit and take the night step-by-step. How did you decide on the restaurant?

JoAnn: My friend picked it, but I looked up the menu online to make sure I knew what I was going to order.

Me: Great! You planned ahead. So what happened when you got to the restaurant?

JoAnn: We were seated right away.

Me: And then?

JoAnn: I don't know, we were just talking.

Me: What about?

JoAnn: Work and kids mostly. And we talked about what we were going to order. She told me she'd been eating healthy all week and was going to order whatever she wanted.

Me: What went through your head when she said that?

JoAnn: Nothing that I can recall.

Me: Slow down and try harder. What were you thinking?

JoAnn: Actually, now that you say that, I did think that I didn't want to order healthy and make her feel bad. But I barely recall thinking that!

Me: Okay, what happened next?

JoAnn: She asked if I wanted to share some calamari. I didn't really want it, but I knew she wanted it and wouldn't get it if I said no. So I said yes and just figured I wouldn't really eat more than one. But I pretty much ate my share.

Me: Okay, so how did you end up ordering a martini instead of a glass of wine?

JoAnn: Well, she ordered one, and I suppose I felt like I needed to follow suit.

Me: So, what happened to your plan to order what you picked out online?

JoAnn: The waiter came and I just panicked. I ordered the fettuccine Alfredo. I would normally never order that.

Me: Okay, so you ordered off plan. What happened next?

JoAnn: Ugh! I kept digging into the bread basket and nearly finished the fettuccine—and it was a lot. I felt sick to my stomach and really frustrated with myself. The whole time I kept saying to myself, "Well you've messed it up now. Back to it tomorrow." But then I just felt so angry with myself afterward.

Me: Here's what I hear you telling me. It sounds like you went with a plan, but your negative self-talk and discomfort with being assertive and sticking to your goals led you to order differently. Even more, once the food was in front of you, your "what-the-heck response" kicked in and you told yourself that eating off plan was what you wanted to do in the moment.

JoAnn: Yep, sounds about right.

Me: Here's what happened. You had a couple of thinking errors going on. First, when your friend told you she was going to eat whatever she wanted, you made an assumption that she would be offended if you ordered healthy. That's mind reading at its finest.

How do you know your healthy habits wouldn't have sparked her to want to eat healthy as well? And second, when you ordered off plan, there were a number of things you could have done to still feel good about your choices, but instead you got caught up in black-and-white thinking, leading you to overeat when you really didn't want to.

JoAnn: So I wasn't really out of control after all. My thoughts made me do it? (She chuckled.)

Me: Yes, that's one way to put it. But more importantly, recognizing that your thought patterns have a way of hindering your success is a great step in understanding how to change your behavior.

What I was doing with JoAnn was Chaining her back through the series of events (links) that led to her ordering off plan at the restaurant. It revealed that some quick but pervasive messages led her to stray from her planned behavior. While you can't always control all your triggers—for example, JoAnn had no control over what her friend ordered and suggested about the calamari—you can control how you react and what choices you make. JoAnn could have advocated for herself by saying something like, "Good for you for eating healthy all week! I'm on the same train, and I'm sticking with a healthy option tonight." This response validates her friend's experience while also advocating for herself. One different choice and her chain of events would have looked very different.

If you suddenly find yourself eating off plan or eating for any other reason than to put fuel in your body, know that a trigger was set off that led to your behavior. Get in the habit of noticing your relationship to food and becoming aware of how and why you choose it. Here is another, more common example of how you can use a different style of Chaining to prevent going off course.

Let's say you're planning on going to a Mexican restaurant with a group of friends. You really like Mexican food and you tend to overeat it, so you decide to look the menu up online and decide what you'll order in advance so you don't have to look at the menu when you get there. All's good. When you arrive, your friends immediately order a couple of plates of nachos—your fave!—and everyone digs in except you. That is, until the buddy sitting next to you passes them right into your hands. You pull four chips from the towering plate and dig in. Now you can't keep your eyes off the cheese-oozing tower of goodness. You can't help but reach for more. Then more again. Before you know it, you ask for a menu and order the pulled pork enchiladas instead of the fish tacos you had planned to order. You say to yourself, "What the heck, I've already ruined my plan to eat healthy tonight." You have entered the mind-set of black-and-white thinking.

In reality, you had many opportunities to break a link in the chain that led to overeating by making a different choice along the way. You could have:

Ordered right away. Placing your entrée order as soon as you sat down would have eliminated the opportunity to change your mind.

Asked the waiter to wrap two of the enchiladas in a take-home bag and only serve you one. Telling yourself you'll only eat half and then asking for a take-home bag doesn't usually work.

Slowly nibbled on your four chips. Savoring the flavors and mindfully paying attention to what you were eating would have helped satiate your desire for the nachos and fortify your resistance for more. (You'll learn how to do this in Step 4.)

Firmly said, "No, thank you, I don't eat nachos" or pushed back your chair so they bypassed you instead of landing in your hands. Letting your buddies know that you seriously don't want nachos anywhere near you would have eliminated the temptation. (You'll learn lots of ways to make this tactic effective in Step 10.)

Not agreed to dine at this particular restaurant. When there is too much temptation and you know the situation will be difficult to control, you always have the choice to opt out, suggest an alternative, or let your friends know that you will only be selecting healthy choices so they don't encourage you.

Cooked a Mexican meal at home. You could have agreed on eating Mexican with your friends, but offered to do the cooking yourself, so you could be totally in charge of the menu.

Each of these links formed the chain of opportunities that could have prevented your unwanted behavior. While you might think that tasting that first nacho is what triggered your behavior, in reality the risk of going awry started when you made the decision to go to a Mexican restaurant with a bunch of friends, which created an environment that was hard to control. If you had acted on any of the previous links, you would likely have had a more favorable outcome. And the sooner in the chain you act, the better. You would have ended the night a satiated and happy guy for not caving in to the temptation to overeat.

CHAINING: FORTIFY THE LINKS TO BETTER BEHAVIOR

Chaining is an exercise that enables you to take complex behaviors and break them down into a series of links in order to better understand why you ended up behaving the way you did. Each link in the chain sets the occasion for the next to take place. Every time you eat off plan or find yourself overeating, chain back through the links you missed that would have broken the chain that led to your unwanted behavior. It will help you better understand how your behaviors occur and the actions you can take to stop them. The following template will get you started. You can use the space provided below or begin the exercise in your journal or notebook. You can download more exercises by looking for the worksheet titled "Chaining" on my Web site, www.elizakingsford.com, and put them in your notebook.

How did I go off plan? What happened?

_____

_____

_____

_____

What was I thinking just before making the decision?

_____

_____

_____

_____

What was I feeling at the time?

_____

_____

_____

_____

Build five chains (actions) that could have changed the outcome:

1. _____
2. _____
3. _____
4. _____
5. _____

What will I do differently next time?

_____
_____
_____
_____

The purpose of Chaining is to condition yourself to become mindful of all the decisions you make around food. People with a Healthy Obsession do it all the time. I do it. I love Mexican food, and I have a hard time resisting chips. As soon as I sit down in my favorite restaurant, I immediately tell the waiter not to bring the complementary chips and salsa. I'm familiar with the menu and know what I should eat, so I never read it. I also love bread, so I always refuse the bread basket in restaurants because I know I will have a hard time stopping at one piece. I don't miss it when I don't taste it. This is easy to do when you learn the many ways you can replace your unsuccessful thinking patterns with more successful ones—which is exactly what you'll be doing in the next two steps, starting with learning how to be more mindful in the way you lead your life (in general) and make your decisions around food (in particular).

MASTER OF WEIGHT LOSS: Debra R.

She Was "Living in Black-and-White Thinking"

I wouldn't call myself a master at weight loss, but I used to be a master at cognitive distortions, so much so that I could have been the poster girl for black-and-white thinking. However, that all started to change in late 2014 when I went to interview Eliza Kingsford for a story I was writing about weight loss.

I'm one of those people who others would describe as "she could stand to lose a few." And it's true. I wasn't really fat, but I definitely wasn't slender. I walked around carrying an extra 15 pounds—give or take a few—for more than 25 years. When Eliza first told me she "can talk anyone into losing weight," my first thought was, "Not me you won't!" And guess what? I was totally wrong.

As I listened to Eliza talk, I realized everything she was saying about how chronic behaviors and triggers sabotage weight-loss efforts made total sense. It was like she was talking about me and my weight-loss efforts for the past 25 years. I had been going on and off diets since I was 19 years old. When I was on, I was starving myself or depriving myself of *something*—carbs, fat, whatever was the fad at the moment. When I was off, I would eat anything or everything. I was constantly living in black-and-white thinking. If I made one slip (that's me she's describing on page 35 ordering the eggs Benedict), I'd figure the entire day was ruined and comfort myself with sinful foods until it was time for bed. The day before I'd start yet another new diet, I'd eat and eat like it was my last meal. And sometimes those diets didn't last for more than a few days.

Several years ago, I just got sick of yo-yoing and decided to find out where I'd end up. Once again, you could've said, "She can stand to lose a few." But not so anymore, because I decided to give Eliza's plan a test-drive. As it turns out, Eliza really *can* talk anybody into losing weight. By listening to what she had to say and following the advice now detailed in this book, I dropped 13 pounds in 5 months. And I didn't "go on a diet." I didn't even change what I eat, because I've always strived to eat healthy. All I did was change my behavior around food.

I got out of the habit of black-and-white thinking and a few other cognitive distortions she describes. I've learned to consider the consequences of my choice *before* I order something and almost always choose, as Eliza likes to say, "What serves me." I never anymore allow a slipup to jeopardize my progress; now, it only makes me strive harder to stay on plan. I stay accountable every single day through MyFitnessPal app, and I make a real effort every day to get in 10,000 steps, even though it's not always that easy. I know without doubt that these new behaviors have allowed me to achieve something I've never done before: Those 13 pounds are still gone, more than a year later.

Find Your Wise Mind through Mindfulness

Psychologist Marsha Linehan, PhD, the creator of Dialectical Behavior Therapy, teaches that at any given time, your mind can be in one of three places: an emotional state, a reasonable state, or a wise state—what I like to call your Wise Mind. Your ultimate goal in achieving Brain-Powered Weight Loss is to spend as much time in your Wise Mind as you can.

Your Emotional Mind is in charge when your thoughts and behaviors are controlled by feelings, which often can be impulsive and intense. When emotions are in charge, your mind can easily distort facts and make you behave irrationally. Reason and logic do not come into play. Things like getting angry at work ("I can't stand working in sales—I'm quitting!"), acting impetuously ("Heck with the gym, let's go get a banana split!"), imagining something has happened to someone who's 30 minutes late ("What if he ran out of gas or, worse, got in an accident?"), and eating a cupcake just because it looks good ("I'm not even hungry, but I can't resist!") are all examples of an Emotional Mind in overdrive.

Think of all the times your Emotional Mind has led you to the cookie jar or to the freezer looking for ice cream. You didn't really want to eat; your Emotional Mind made you do it. Every cognitive distortion you learned about in Step 3 comes about when your Emotional Mind rules your life.

Your Reasonable Mind rules when you are task oriented, thinking logically, paying attention to your surroundings, making fact-based decisions, and consistently being intentional about your behavior—like you should be when you're driving a car. When your Reasonable Mind is in charge, you are ruled by facts, reason, logic, and pragmatics. There is no place in your decision for emotion; values and feelings are not important. Your unhappiness at work becomes, "I can't quit until I find another job." Forgoing the gym becomes,

"There is never a reason for missing the gym." Your worry over waiting for someone becomes, "He's always late." Being offered the cupcake is immediately rebuked with, "There is no nutritional value in a cupcake."

A Reasonable Mind might sound like a good place to be, but when you let it rule, life can become much too rigid. When you spend too much time in your Reasonable Mind, you're devoid of emotion. You act or react without considering the circumstances or consequences. For example, you find out your son didn't do his homework like you'd asked, so you slap your hand on the counter and respond, "You're grounded all weekend!" But where's the context? Where's the feeling? It's quite possible he didn't do his homework because he didn't understand it and was too embarrassed to ask for help. If you would have injected a little emotion first, you'd have asked, "Can you tell me why you didn't do your homework? Do you need help with it?"

If you lived solely in your Reasonable Mind, you'd find it hard to make and keep friends or bond in a loving relationship, because relationships are fostered through emotion. You'd find it difficult to experience joy and happiness. You'd get no pleasure out of eating and would consider food as nothing more than fuel for your body. You'd never be at peace with yourself because you've handcuffed yourself to rigidity, and most likely you'd eventually rebel—"This vegan diet could take me forever to lose weight. I want out!"

Thankfully, the Wise Mind emerges when these two minds overlap. It looks like this:

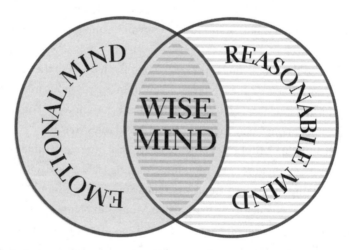

It takes the best of both your Emotional Mind and your Reasonable Mind to merge as your Wise Mind.

You are most authentic when you are in your Wise Mind. Being in your Wise Mind means you are thinking at your best, often responding to what is commonly called your "gut feeling." You instinctively feel the difference between right and wrong. You intuitively recognize the difference between your emotions and your reasoning, and you have the ability to make the best decision and follow through, using a little of both. The desire to quit your job on the spot might instead look like, "So, I didn't make any sales today, but overall I am really successful at selling." The urge to skip the gym becomes, "Skipping the gym just because I don't feel like going is not a great choice for me." Worrying while waiting for someone to show up becomes, "I might as well work and make use of this time while I'm waiting." The tempting cupcake becomes, "It looks good, but I don't need or want one."

When you're in your Wise Mind, you are centered and grounded, and have your life and thoughts in balance. You are not making decisions based solely on emotions; neither are you devoid of them. When you are in your Wise Mind, you can refocus the urge for some ice cream by reminding yourself how crappy it's going to make you feel afterward and how frustrated you'll be with yourself for eating it. Or, if you are making an intentional choice to eat ice cream, it's your Wise Mind that gives you the ability to accept your decision and get yourself back on plan—not tomorrow or Monday or on January 1, but *now*.

Living in your Wise Mind does not mean your life is always going to be easy. It does not mean that losing weight and maintaining your weight loss will be a breeze. However, living in your Wise Mind will give you the ability to handle life and whatever struggles enter it with intention, acceptance, and nonjudgmental awareness.

If you've been in a constant struggle with your weight, most likely you spend too much time leading with your Emotional Mind and possibly too little time making decisions with your Reasonable Mind. For example, it's your Emotional Mind that sends you into a tailspin that leads to an all-out binge because you went off plan by drinking a milkshake, whereas your Wise Mind allows you to stop, slow down, and check in: "That milkshake tasted great, but I don't feel very good about drinking it. I'm getting right back on track, where I know I'll feel good eating foods that are in line with my goals." There's no black-and-white thinking, no disqualifying the positive, no mental filtering, no mind reading. Rather, you know you can't change what just happened, *but* it's totally up to you what happens next. You are being nonjudg-mental ("Shakes happen!"), aware ("I can't change what I did, but I can control what I do next"), and intentional ("I'm back on track").

We all have the ability to learn to live mostly in our Wise Minds. The surest way to get there is through learning the practice of mindfulness, an effective and increasingly studied skill for resolving an array of issues, food being one of them. It's an integral part of the brain-powered plan because being mindful means you are thinking with your Wise Mind—which brings me to Brain-Powered Pointer No. 8:

> Practicing mindfulness helps you
> find your Wise Mind.

Mindfulness is one of the most important skills you are going to learn and one I encourage you to embrace and use often. Consider it your number one go-to tool for changing the way you think about and behave around food.

MINDFULNESS:
THE PLAYBOOK TO A WISER MIND

Mindfulness is a highly effective form of attention-control training that teaches us how to focus and be present in the here and now and take each moment as it comes. It allows us to experience life as we are living it with awareness, clarity, and acceptance in the absence of judgment.

Mindfulness is an ages-old Eastern practice introduced into Western cul-ture more than 30 years ago by Jon Kabat-Zinn, PhD. In his seminal book *Wherever You Go, There You Are*, Dr. Kabat-Zinn calls mindfulness "the art of conscious living."

Mindfulness is the antithesis of multitasking. When you are being mind-ful, you can't listen to your kids talking about their school day while checking your to-do list, because your attention is solely focused on what your children are telling you. When you are being mindful, you aren't eating your lunch while checking your e-mails, because you're completely paying attention to the enjoyment of the food. When you are being mindful, you can't jump to conclusions or initiate any of the other cognitive distortions that dominate your life. When you are being mindful, you won't automatically find yourself in front of the freezer with a pint of ice cream in your hand because you are always in touch with what, when, where, why, and how you eat.

Mindfulness is integral to changing our thought patterns and the behaviors they create because paying attention to how we genuinely experience daily life is the foundation of change. It allows us to understand our feelings, thoughts, and emotions and how they interact with our world. It helps break the self-perpetuating cycle of cognitive distortions that cause us to overeat and thwart our ability to stay on track. Practicing attention control works because it gives us the ability to pause in the moment (passing by a tray of cupcakes) and then *respond* ("Thanks just the same, but I'm not hungry"), rather than *react* ("Just got to have one!"). Being mindful reminds us that we have choices. We can choose to either turn to food or deal with a situation without involving food.

Both Western medical and psychological sciences have embraced mindfulness as an effective tool because hundreds of scientific studies conducted over the last few decades have found it increases overall health and helps combat a long list of medical and psychological issues, including overcoming the inability to lose weight and sustain weight loss. Specific to overweight and the issues that impede weight loss, practicing mindfulness has been found to help:

- Strengthen our ability to regulate our emotions
- Foster positive thoughts and emotions
- Increase happiness and improve mood
- Ameliorate uncontrollable eating and preoccupation with food
- Decrease an interest in eating unhealthy foods
- Shield us from stress and emotional eating
- Reduce dependence on the triggers that cause overeating and binge eating
- Improve an awareness of satiety
- Decrease anxiety, anger, depression, fatigue, and tension
- Decrease negative thinking and avoidance behaviors
- Increase our sense of well-being
- Improve resilience, focus, and learning

All these remarkable mental changes are possible because repeating a practice over and over can change and create new neural pathways in the brain, a process known as neuroplasticity. For example, one study, conducted at Harvard University, found the area of the brain involved in emotional regulation called the insula grew stronger in people who practiced mindfulness. Another study, conducted at the University of Pittsburgh, found that practicing mindfulness thickens the prefrontal cortex, the area of the brain that controls the high-level skills known as executive function, and shrinks the amygdala, the area of the brain that initiates stress.

These studies were not conducted on monks dedicated to a life of meditation in a monastery, but on regular folks like you and me who participated in a formal 6- or 8-week course in which they learned mindfulness through meditation.

MINDFULNESS MEDITATION

Meditation takes little thought—and that's the challenge. Our minds are typically racing with lots of thoughts like cars speeding over, under, and through the busy superhighways that traverse a large city. When you meditate, it's more like meandering alone down a quiet country road.

Some people have a knee-jerk reaction to the idea of meditation. If you're one of them, just put the word aside—don't get lost in it. The type of meditation known as mindfulness meditation does not involve chanting, prayer, or adopting mantras. It is neither spiritual nor religious in nature. Mindfulness meditation is simply the practice of training the brain to be aware, nonjudgmentally and on purpose. Mindfulness won't make life easier, but it will help you make managing its many challenges easier. It won't make weight loss easier, but it will help you stick with your commitment. It may even help you achieve long-term weight control. Studies suggest that people who practice mindfulness meditation typically are at a healthier weight.

Attention training breaks the cycle of autopilot, the time you spend just going along with your day, unconsciously popping jelly beans in your mouth, for example, rather than making a conscious or intentional choice such as "I don't want or desire candy." As you practice focusing your attention, you will begin to become more aware of the unconscious thoughts that influence your behavior. You will be able to pause and reflect on what's happening in the moment and notice the unconscious mental habits that have been driving your decisions and choices. As you build the skill to recognize these habits, it will become easier to take them in a healthier direction. You'll notice you can handle change better, you'll be less reactive, and you'll be able to accept yourself for who you are. You will see life with more clarity.

Practicing mindfulness by focusing on your breathing sounds simple enough, but it requires effort and discipline because the forces that work against you—your cognitive distortions, automatic thoughts and habits—are tenacious. It takes time for unconscious thoughts and habits to subside, so mindfulness needs to be nurtured. However, studies show that daily repetitive practice for 6 to 8 weeks can result in recognizable benefits.

You can learn to be mindful without meditation, though meditating itself is a proven and profoundly helpful tool. As you train your attention on your breath, you'll become more aware of your thoughts and how they run through your mind during the day.

Mental Resilience Technique: S-T-O-P and Let Go of That Thought

Your day's not going your way and it's stressing you out. . . . You're angry with your kids again for not cleaning up their rooms. . . . Your boss is, well, a jerk, or at least you think so. . . . Whenever a situation erupts that can trigger overeating or the berating self-talk that tugs at your emotions, do this: Pause, breathe, and then respond by employing the mindfulness practice that goes by the acronym STOP:

S—Stop what you are doing.

T—Take a deep breath or two.

O—Observe your feelings and your thoughts.

P—Proceed with intention, *choosing* what you will say or do next.

Pausing can stop a knee-jerk reaction that can manifest an untenable situation. It allows you to respond and take a different path: "What could I do differently? What would my Wise Mind do or say?"

FOLLOW YOUR BREATH

Mindfulness meditation is simple in concept. Its power comes from its practice—concentrating for several minutes or longer on a single object, the breath being the most common. You can integrate mindfulness meditation into your life by simply stopping throughout the day to become aware of your breathing. While most of the studies on the benefits of mindfulness focused on 30 minutes of meditation, experts say you can experience positive changes by practicing for 5 seconds, 5 minutes, 15 minutes, or longer each day over the course of several weeks. The ideal setting puts you in a quiet place without distraction or with only pleasing natural sounds in the background, such as water moving or birds chirping. This is a good way to start. Ultimately, your goal will be to have the ability to practice mindfulness meditation in any setting because you will be able to focus your mind amid distraction.

You can do it sitting down, standing up, lying down (just don't fall asleep), or even while you're walking. You are not trying to still the mind. Rather, you are trying in a very gentle way to keep your mind focused on a single something: your breath. Your mind will wander—it's to be expected—but each time it does, gently bring it back. As you continue in the practice, moments of wandering will get shorter and you'll be able to stay focused on your breath for longer periods.

When starting your meditation, observe how you are feeling in the moment. Don't try to change anything. Fully accept how you are feeling. Slowly breathe in through the nose in your normal way and out through your mouth, keeping your mind focused on each breath. Just breathe in and out. In, out. When thoughts enter your mind, and they inevitably will, just notice them. Say to yourself something like, "Oh, I've deviated from my breath. Bring it back," and refocus on your breathing. Do not judge your thoughts, good or bad. Your goal is to notice that the thoughts arise but to not follow them. For example, if you find yourself thinking that you need to go to the grocery store, your goal is to recognize you are thinking about it but avoid making a shopping list. Don't follow the thoughts, bring your mind back to your breath. Allow yourself to be who you are and accept what is exactly as it is.

That's all there is to it. You can learn the skill on your own. All you have to do is keep at it every day or, even better, several times a day. If you feel you need assistance, there are several smartphone apps you can use (just search "mindfulness meditation apps"); you can sign up for a formal class, if one is offered in your community; or you can listen to CDs or other audios that teach it.

THE ART OF BEING NONJUDGMENTAL

Paying attention to how we experience our daily lives is the foundation for change. It allows us to become familiar with our thoughts, feelings, and emotions as we interact with the world around us. Rather than react—"Oh no, you broke my good china, you careless child!"—we learn to respond: "It's just a plate. I know it wasn't intentional." Rather than reacting with the calamity of "I can't believe I ate all that," you respond with, "It was just a slip at one meal, and now I'm moving on in my health quest."

Reactions are judgments often triggered by thoughts or trying situations. They escalate our stress levels—"This should have never happened!" But it did, and no amount of chocolate cake can change that. Life can never be different than it is in the particular moment we are living it. Yet, when things don't go our way, we reactively get upset or stressed out or lapse into cognitive distortions. But things are as they are. You cannot undo what just happened; the only thing you can control is what you do next.

Mindfulness is often defined as "being fully aware of what is happening in the present moment *without judgment.*" Judgments, either good or bad, that we attach to the situations in our lives are what cause our emotions and behaviors to take us in a direction that does not serve us. For example, there is a difference between being stalled in a traffic jam and fuming, "I'm going to be late for work," and fretting about how much trouble you will be in, and simply acknowledging you're stuck in traffic and will probably be late for work—"I'm in the same boat as everybody else in this jam." Worrying about being in trouble is fortune-telling. How do you know? No amount of angst and anxiety can change the traffic, but it can certainly change your mood and, as you've learned, your behavior!

Changing problematic thoughts and behaviors means recognizing the difference between clear thoughts—"I should call ahead and let work know I'll be late"—and being judgmental—"Some a&$hole is holding up traffic!" One of the ways mindfulness teaches this is through a practice called Loving Kindness.

Practice Loving Kindness

Loving Kindness is a mindfulness practice designed to heal difficult emotions and replace them with healing love and acceptance. It helps increase our sense of love and compassion, first for ourselves, then for our loved ones, and then for all the other people in our world, especially those who tend to make our lives difficult. It helps protect us from developing and holding on to anger, hostility, and being judgmental.

Loving Kindness meditation is one of the first things I'll prescribe to someone who is struggling with a negative body image and a lot of self-doubt. As the late Martin Luther King Jr. famously said, "Hate cannot drive out hate, only love can do that. Darkness cannot drive out darkness, only light can do that." The same is true for you. You cannot hate yourself into loving yourself. You cannot hate your body into being the body you want. You can, however, learn compassion for yourself.

Practicing Loving Kindness is like saying a prayer, repeating to yourself kind and loving words and wishes for the sake of yourself and others. Here's how to go about it:

- Select a person to whom you want to direct Loving Kindness. It's best to start with yourself, but if this is too difficult, choose someone you love. Do not start with someone causing difficulty in your life.

- Comfortably sit, stand, or lie down and begin breathing deeply and slowly. Open the palms of your hands and gently bring that person to mind.

- Recite a set of positive wishes you want to convey, such as "May I be healthy, may I be at peace, may I be happy." Repeat the phrases slowly, focusing on the meaning of each word as you say it to yourself. If distractions enter your mind (and they will at first), gently pull your thoughts back. Continue until you feel yourself immersed in Loving Kindness.

- Gradually work your way through your circle of people, starting with your most beloved, then your friends, then those who make your life difficult, your enemies, and finally all beings. Radiate your Loving Kindness with words directed at each—"May I be happy, may John be happy . . ."

- Practice daily.

FLAVOR YOUR FOOD WITH MINDFULNESS

We all have to eat. It is a basic requirement of life. Yet, all too frequently we go about it in the wrong way: We do it mindlessly. We grab breakfast while packing the kids' lunches and sneaking peaks at the morning show. We grab lunch on the run, and often eat dinner in a flood of conversation with the evening news in the background. We go through the drive-thru and eat while we drive, text, or play games on our smartphones. It's called mindless eating, a bad habit that works against you in many ways.

When you eat mindlessly, you risk eating too much and miss the important internal cues that say, "That was satisfying, but I've had enough." You also miss out on one of the true pleasures in life: *enjoying* food. However, when you eat mind*fully*, your focus is only on the act of eating and the appreciation of the food—how it looks, tastes, smells, and feels. It allows you to appreciate food more and be satisfied with less because you are being attentive to your goals. When you take the time to actually taste the food, you fulfill the desire to eat.

Being mindful means focusing on one thing: what you are doing here and now. Doing one thing at a time with intention and focus is important when you are eating because it guarantees your Wise Mind is in charge, keeping you from straying beyond the eating boundaries you have set for yourself. When you are mindful, you engage all your senses in your eating, restaurant, and food-buying decisions. Think of all the times you eat only because something looks or smells good. When you are mindful, however, you can resist moving in this direction. Being mindful means being intentional about the foods you select when shopping and what you choose to cook at home or order in a restaurant.

Eating mindfully from meal to meal and day to day is a learned skill. Like anything else, it gets easier and more instinctual with practice. Here's how to go about it.

Limit distractions. Eating mindfully does not mean eating in solitude all the time. That wouldn't be any fun. However, you should avoid distractions when eating with others. At home, make it a rule to turn off televisions, music, and other background noise. All phones should be off-limits in eating spaces. Discipline family members and close friends to not talk over others, and put volatile topics of conversation off limits.

Bring your full attention to the food. Eat in small bites, chew slowly, and rest your utensils on the table between bites. Notice the sight, sound, smell, touch, and taste of the food in front of you. If you are dining with others, rest between bites and bring your full attention to that experience, too.

Pay attention to your thoughts and emotions. Notice when negative self-talk is dominating your food choices when shopping and preparing meals, and when it is influencing serving size. Check in with yourself before taking a second helping by asking, "Am I hungry? Have I eaten enough to satiate myself?"

Pause often while eating. Pay attention to your body cues. Stop when you are no longer hungry, rather than eating until you feel full. There is a difference! There is no need to eat the plate clean.

Notice your food habits. Pause before making all food choices. Without self-judgment about what has happened before, make intentional decisions about the foods you buy and plan to eat at your next meal.

Avoid negative self-talk if you don't succeed. Habitual behaviors are difficult, but not impossible, to break. If you don't succeed today, give yourself credit for your successes, however small. Plan a better strategy for tomorrow.

MASTER OF WEIGHT LOSS: Jonathan Q.

"Mindfulness Has Increased My Joy of Life"

I know as well as just about anybody what a struggle it is to lose weight and keep it off, because I've lost and regained a combined total of more than 200 pounds over the last 12 years. That's almost half my life.

My weight gain began when I was in fourth grade, right around the time my parents split up and eventually divorced. I was told my eating patterns may have been an emotional response, but whatever the reason, they stuck around and became ingrained in habit. By the time I was 13, my parents sat me down and announced they were sending me to this camp called Wellspring. At the time, I was 270 pounds and just under 5-foot-10. I was a *big* boy. At first I resisted, as many 13-year-olds would.

As it turned out, I had an incredible time and lost almost 40 pounds.

Only here's what I didn't quite get at first: Anybody can lose weight by exercising and following a planned healthy diet, but it takes a lifestyle change to make it stick. It took me four incredible summers at Wellspring to really figure that out.

My last summer before college, I went to a Wellspring camp that was more fitness focused. I took up running and weight training for the first time. I was also playing hockey again, something I loved as a little kid but was forced to give up because I gained so much weight I couldn't physically keep up. That summer I turned into a new me. I lost 60 pounds. Entering college, I was over 6 feet tall and weighed about 190 pounds, looking and feeling better than I ever had in my life. Fresh out of camp, I was extra-vigilant with my program and managed to avoid the freshman 15 that everyone else was gaining. I kept the weight off until my senior year, when I put on 40 pounds, partly due to breaking my foot but also because of the conscious decision to let loose and ditch my self-monitoring. It took time and hard work to get the weight off after college, but by then I had identified an important concept: Whenever I fell off the self-monitoring bandwagon, I was less in control of my dietary and exercise choices and weight gain usually followed.

The thing that stuck with me after four summers at camp is that you have complete control over yourself and your decisions. You can make an unhealthy decision one moment, but you can also make a healthy decision the next moment and just move forward. It became apparent to me that at the times in my life when I self-monitored, I made more of those healthy, informed decisions, and when I didn't self-monitor I didn't take accountability for the less healthy decisions I made. I was dishonest with myself and would rationalize why I made those choices. It felt like a million people told me a billion times that self-monitoring was *that* important. For example, when I didn't self-monitor, I could rush through a full bag of tortilla chips without even realizing it. When I wasn't self-monitoring, I became a mindless eater. I think this stems from bad habits I formed as a kid. At home when I was young, the unhealthy snacks were always hidden and locked away from me. I'd go on a mission to find them. When I did, I'd just eat and eat. When I'd gain too much, I'd get back on plan. That's not the way it's supposed to work!

By the summer of 2015, I returned to Wellspring, this time as a counselor. It's something I always wanted to do because the camp has had such a profound impact on my life. It was at this time that Eliza Kingsford started to incorporate mindfulness into Wellspring's behavioral therapy program. I decided to take up meditation after my first summer as a counselor. I downloaded the app called Headspace and gave mindfulness a try. I loved it and started to make meditation and the practice of mindfulness a habit. It was the turning point for me; it changed my life.

Even though I am not a particularly anxious person, mindfulness slows me down and allows me to think more clearly and with more ease. Using mindfulness in a calm, knowledgeable manner allows me to make informed decisions about eating, exercise, relationships, and most everything else in my life. I've come to realize that self-monitoring *is* being mindful. The two are intertwined. Being mindful keeps me engaged in self-monitoring and prevents me from straying too far from my goals. It's now habitual that I eat mindfully, appreciating each bite, living in the moment. In the past when I would go off the self-monitoring bandwagon, I would eat mindlessly and in bulk. I wouldn't truly enjoy my food. When you eat mindfully, you enjoy each bite, something my old habits never allowed me to do.

Today, I'm back to 190 pounds. I'm fit and feel more in control of my health and well-being than I ever have. I credit mindfulness meditation for making this happen. Mindfulness has increased my joy of life. Meditation has helped me identify habits and patterns worth working on and changing in the same way self-monitoring has. And on top of that, I've got this newfound love for life and appreciation for every moment that I hope I can share with the world.

I'm 25 and still trying to figure things out. I'm not sure where I will land next, though I've got some ideas. When I was a kid, I didn't really get it that behavioral therapy, habit change, and healthy habit formation are key to long-term sustainability. Mindfulness has helped me become aware of the power behind those methods. I believe mindfulness will continue to make me a happier and healthier person.

Learn Your Dealing Skills—Then Use Them

Dealing Skills are a set of mental tools and exercises designed to train your brain to drown out the voice that is your Emotional Mind and heal your relationship with food. They create the bridge of change that will take you from a life of struggling with overeating and overweight to one focused on healthy living and healthy eating. They are the tools you are going to use time and again to wash away the cognitive distortions that unconsciously flood your mind and replace them with conscious decisions seeded with mindfulness and a healthy focus. In essence, all the exercises in this book are Dealing Skills, but the ones you are going to learn in this step are focused on these agents of change:

- Easing your struggle with regulating your emotions, especially around food

- Learning how to better tolerate situations and circumstances that drive poor eating choices and the desire to overeat or binge

- Improving your personal effectiveness skills when dealing with others in ways that better serve you, your weight-loss goals, and your weight control needs

In order to get your mind in the right space to use these Dealing Skills, consciously try to approach your life as it is right now with what's called Radical Acceptance. This means accepting your current relationship and struggles with food without judgment. "I recognize and accept that I have gained 30 pounds and am on this journey to lose it permanently," not "I can't believe I gained back all 30 pounds and now I have to do all this stuff." Or "I recognize and accept that I overeat every time I go to a Mexican restaurant because the

Learn the Skills of Acceptance and Change

Many people struggle with weight loss because their minds are so conflicted about themselves. They hate how they look and desire to change, yet they can't seem to make it happen. It's like they want to ignore who they are until a wish or mental image about themselves becomes reality: "That's what I desire, but until then, I'm not who I want to be."

This kind of thinking only gets in the way of your goals because it keeps you in a constant state of negativity *until* you reach the state you desire sometime in the future. It does not serve you. It creates an internal conflict that perpetuates living in cognitive distortions.

The way to move forward with strength and conviction is by accepting and loving who you are now while at the same time wanting to change who you are. Like yes and no, left and right, back and forth, right and wrong, these opposites need the other to exist. There would be no left without right. No right without wrong. It is possible to work on these two opposing states at the same time. You can work on this by accepting and using this affirmation:

I am willing to love and accept who I am, and I am willing to change.

food is hard to resist," not "I eat like a pig every time I go to a Mexican restaurant because I can't control myself around the food." You gained 30 pounds, so believe it. Mexican restaurants are a trigger, so accept it. They are your current reality.

Accepting your reality without judgment will allow you to access your Wise Mind when practicing your Dealing Skills. It's the best place to be. Remember, you can't change what got you to the weight you are not happy with now. No amount of self-deprecation or berating yourself over it is going to help you or take you back in time. Instead, treat yourself differently. Radical Acceptance is about pushing through those feelings of anger, frustration, and disappointment and instead fiercely accepting where you are right now, just as you are, without judgment or blame. Sound impossible? It's not. That's why it's radical! Now let's get started.

CREATING A NEW INTERNAL DIALOGUE

Have you ever been caught up in this kind of thinking?

I dieted hard all week; I SHOULD have lost more weight.

I CAN'T go out to dinner with you this week because I NEED to lose two more pounds by Saturday.

I CAN'T go to happy hour because I HAVE to go to the gym instead.

I CAN'T eat fried chicken like the rest of you because I MUST eat only a salad.

Should, can't, need, have, and *must* are all one-word diet traps. They are nothing but negative extremes and absolutes that don't demand any action. Rather, they constantly remind you that you're trapped, you're miserable, and you can't wait "until this diet is over" so you can get your life back again. This kind of thinking has only one outcome: self-defeat. The extremes and absolutes that create your mental chatter are the catalysts of what's called the Lethargy Cycle of Self-Defeating Thoughts, and it goes like this:

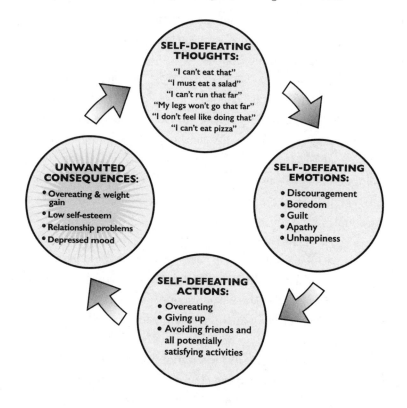

You sink deeper into the self-conviction that you cannot lose weight and the negative emotions that accompany it, which leads to more self-defeating thoughts as the cycle continues.

Nothing pleasant can come out of self-defeating thoughts. All the I can'ts, I musts, and I shoulds that you typically attach to the traditional act of dieting only lead to self-defeating emotions, which lead to self-defeating actions that result in lethargic consequences, sinking you deeper and deeper into an unmotivated state of paralysis—"It's unfair I have to work so hard to look like my thin friends when they don't have to deprive themselves." It's another reason why diets don't work, which brings me to Brain-Powered Pointer No. 9:

> **It's difficult to lose weight when you feel like you're depriving yourself of fun and pleasure all the time.**

Now, let's change the above sample internal dialogue just a little and see how it feels to be out of the habit of thinking and acting in extremes and absolutes.

"I dieted hard all week; I should have lost more weight" becomes "I ate according to my goals all week, and that makes me feel empowered. I know I'm making progress." You've erased the defeatist word *diet* from your vocabulary and know your new proactive approach to eating only healthy, nourishing foods will bring lots of positive results.

"I can't go out to dinner with you this week because I need to lose two more pounds by Saturday" becomes "I'd love to go out to dinner with you. If you don't mind, let me pick the restaurant." You are no longer putting life on hold while trying another fad diet. When your path is toward a healthier lifestyle, life simply goes on as usual, bringing your healthy decisions along with it. And it's exciting because you know this path will lead to you feeling and looking so much better. Offering to pick the restaurant ensures that you can be in control of what you eat.

"I can't go to happy hour because I have to go to the gym instead" becomes "I'll catch up with you at the bar later because I want to go to the gym." You'll feel great after an aerobic workout, which has now become your choice and not your punishment. You know that working out will give you more energy, and you'll be glad you did something healthy for yourself before going out with friends—a real boost of self-confidence!

"I can't eat fried chicken like the rest of you because I must eat only a salad" becomes "I don't want fried chicken; I much prefer grilled chicken." Your conviction—"I don't" instead of "I can't"—is powerfully persuasive. In fact, one study found that unspecific postponements, such as declaring "I don't want" to a food, reduces the desire for the food, both in the present moment and gradually over time.

How to Hone Your Dealing Skills

Dealing Skills are your toolbox to change. I recommend you try out all of them, then concentrate on using the tools that are most authentic to resolving your particular thinking errors and personal struggles with overeating, unhealthy eating, and exercise. The more you practice them, the more they will become automatic and an everyday part of life.

The foundation for retraining your brain is grounded in the three Rs: Recognize, Replace, and Repeat.

RECOGNIZE. Slow yourself down so you can recognize what is taking place at any particular moment in time that jeopardizes your healthy eating and exercise goals and puts you at risk of overeating or bingeing. The earlier you can catch yourself and recognize the cues that get you into trouble with food, the faster you can respond and head off the potential damage. For example, let's say you didn't get enough sleep, and you know from experience that lack of sleep makes you grumpy and shakes your resolve to choose healthy food— "I didn't sleep well again last night, and the only thing that's going to help get me through this day is a caramel Frappuccino." Recognize when this mental shakedown is taking place and replace it with a positive counter thought immediately.

REPLACE. Immediately replace your sabotaging thought or event with a relevant Dealing Skill or Skills. For example, you can respond to your lack of sleep by replacing your negative thought with a positive affirmation: "Each healthy choice I make gets me closer to finding my Healthy Obsession." Say it, even if in the moment you don't believe it. Saying it will help make it so.

REPEAT. Change is all about consistency, consistency, consistency. Practice makes permanent. Every time your mind strays into a negative distortion or problematic emotion, draw back to your Wise Mind with positive counter thoughts. Every. Single. Time. The more you do this, the more you'll do it!

LETTING GO OF EXTREMES AND ABSOLUTES

To find out how much your life is governed by thinking in absolutes, I'd like you to spend one full day—tomorrow, preferably—consciously living without them. Take note when you find any of these words governing your actions:

- Should
- Should not
- Have to
- Can't
- Need to
- Ought to
- Must
- Must not

These are words that lead to self-defeating thoughts. As you go through your day and catch yourself saying or thinking one of these words, mindfully stop, pause, reflect on what is happening, then rephrase. For example:

> **Self-Defeating Thought:** Everyone at the table is enjoying the bread basket. I want some bread so badly, but I *can't* have any because it is off-limits on this stupid diet. It's not fair that they eat it and don't gain weight.
>
> **Positive Counter Thought:** Eating bread does not serve me. I have choices, and I choose not to eat bread.

Now in the space below, write down the thoughts that occur to you during the day and frequently occur in your life, and rephrase them into powerful convictions. There is space here for 10, but if you prefer, you can write them in your journal or get the worksheet "Self-Defeating Thoughts/Positive Counter Thoughts" for your notebook by going to my Web site, www.elizakingsford.com.

1. **Self-Defeating Thought:** _____
   Positive Counter Thought: _____
2. **Self-Defeating Thought:** _____
   Positive Counter Thought: _____

3. Self-Defeating Thought: _____

   Positive Counter Thought: _____

4. Self-Defeating Thought: _____

   Positive Counter Thought: _____

5. Self-Defeating Thought: _____

   Positive Counter Thought: _____

6. Self-Defeating Thought: _____

   Positive Counter Thought: _____

7. Self-Defeating Thought: _____

   Positive Counter Thought: _____

8. Self-Defeating Thought: _____

   Positive Counter Thought: _____

9. Self-Defeating Thought: _____

   Positive Counter Thought: _____

10. Self-Defeating Thought: _____

   Positive Counter Thought: _____

This is an important exercise meant to help you change the thought patterns that intrude with your weight loss and make you lose sight of your weight-management goals. The more you consciously become aware of all the can'ts, musts, and shouldn'ts you impose on yourself, the more cognizant you'll become of their existence. You'll see them for what they really are— self-imposed rigidity that's bound to backfire sooner or later. As you practice changing your negative reactions into positive responses, you'll gradually and naturally start behaving in accordance.

Often, however, our problem behaviors go much deeper than digging into a bag of potato chips or throwing out a salad because you bullied yourself with so many can'ts and shouldn'ts that you had to have a Reuben sandwich. We also use thoughts against ourselves in ways that blemish our self-confidence, self-worth, and self-esteem. These types of mental patterns are even more intrusive on our weight-loss efforts because the thoughts we use against ourselves tend to become so automatic that we don't even recognize them.

TAKE THE AUTOMATIC OUT OF YOUR THOUGHTS

Automatic thoughts are instantaneous, habitual, and unconscious self-talk we often use against ourselves and often blow out of proportion. These words, phrases, and notions are powerful because they charge our emotions and influence our behavior. They also can be cunning because we don't always realize what we are saying to ourselves—these thoughts are that ingrained and automatic. Our subsequent actions, however, are real and have real consequences. For example, you always wear a cover-up or baggy shirt over your bathing suit at the beach and never take it off, even when it's deadly hot,

Learn the Skill of Diversion

Something is happening that has you emotionally strung out: You are fighting with your spouse again for going out drinking after work. You hear rumors about downsizing at the place you work. Your child swore at you and ran out of the house. You have to go on another boring vacation with your in-laws.

When life doesn't go the way you want it to, the mind of a habitual dieter more often than not responds by turning to food. That only adds more emotional baggage and makes a stressful situation worse. It also heightens your risk of falling into the Lethargy Cycle of Self-Defeating Thoughts. However, you can accept reality and face it with this fact: Life is never going to always go the way you want it to. Accept it and become fluent at tolerating distressing situations without using food or falling into other problem behaviors. That only makes a bad situation worse. Instead, treat yourself to something better.

There are times when you'll need to distract yourself, times when you'll need to soothe yourself, and times when you'll need to improve the moment. Be at the ready by having a plan for all three. For example, you can distract yourself by calling a good friend you know who can always make you laugh. Or, if you love gardening, you can lose yourself working in your yard. You can soothe yourself by buying flowers, listening to music, getting a massage, or doing whatever brings you pleasure. You can improve any moment by doing mindful meditation, going for a walk, or hugging your kids or dog. Think about your own life and the things that because that voice in your head says, "I'm so embarrassed by my huge thighs." Or you work through lunch and eat at your desk because you think, "Everybody stares at how much I eat because I'm so fat." Or you avoid shopping for clothes because you believe, "I look awful in *everything*." Or you're getting dressed to go to work and find your size 8 pencil skirt no longer fits and you think, "One cheeseburger and there I go again; I'll never be able to keep my weight off," and by lunch you don't understand why you're eating a hoagie instead of a salad.

None of these thoughts are consciously going through your head, but they are subconsciously *in* your head making you behave the way you do. They do

make you happy. Write them down here, or download "Diversion Skills Practice" from my Web site, www.elizakingsford.com, for your journal or notebook. Get in the habit of making them your go-to diversions.

MY BEST DISTRACTIONS:

1. _____

2. _____

3. _____

MY BEST SELF-SOOTHERS:

1. _____

2. _____

3. _____

MY BEST WAYS OF ENHANCING A MOMENT:

1. _____

2. _____

3. _____

nothing for your self-esteem, which puts you in the Lethargy Cycle of Self-Defeating Thoughts, which consequently leads to overeating and/or abandoning your weight-loss goals. Think about it: Would you really prefer to sweat in your baggy cover-up than be comfortable, eat all alone in a cavernous room than in the cafeteria with your teammates, or never shop for something fun to wear? Do you really want to abandon that pencil skirt for good?

We have a tendency to say things over and over to ourselves so often, we can convince ourselves that what we think is true. For example, when you exclaim "I'm starving!" (though you're actually not) as you walk to lunch with your buddies from work, you're more apt to *act* like you're starving and impulsively order what sounds irresistible instead of what's healthy. Saying "It's freezing outside!" (no, it's just a little cold) immediately shuts down the possibility that you'll take a walk today. Saying "I hate broccoli" puts too high a premium on broccoli when you should be saving your hate for such things as terrorism or bigotry. Thinking your thighs are huge is enough to make it real—in *your* mind. Believing that one cheeseburger can make a skirt too tight is deflating enough to abandon all the hard work you've done up to this point.

It's tough to pursue any goal when you're down on yourself all or most of the time, but it's even more difficult to pursue your weight-loss goals because your food choices are so intertwined with how you feel from day to day. From my experience with people I counsel, I say it's almost impossible, *unless* you learn to take the automatic out of your thoughts. The way to do it is to consciously challenge them, which is something we seldom or never do. Rather, we are more prone to look for evidence to prove our thoughts are right-on than we are to spend the time to disprove them. Now, hold that thought for a moment. . . . Trying to defend your own negativity doesn't make any sense at all! To turn these thoughts into favorable behaviors, you need to challenge them, which brings me to Brain-Powered Pointer No. 10:

Challenging automatic thoughts requires practice, practice, practice.

As you practice bringing more balance to your thoughts, you'll begin to see a marked improvement in your self-compassion and self-confidence, which will allow you to respond ("I'm making slow but steady progress") instead of react ("I look horrible"). The next exercise will show you how.

AUTOMATIC THOUGHTS CHALLENGE

This exercise is designed to help you play detective by examining your own thoughts. Find about 30 minutes in your day to set this in motion. You'll have to find a quiet place where you can sit and examine your actions, so you can relate them to a thought. Here's how this exercise unfolds:

1. You start by stating the thought and your belief about the thought.
2. You look for evidence to support it—the real facts.
3. Lastly, you challenge it by modifying the belief.

Because you are starting out with prejudice—that is, you believe yourself—you must intentionally make yourself impartial. To help yourself approach this exercise with neutrality, ask yourself these questions:

- Is your thought based on your opinion alone, or is it based on what other people have said or what you believe they have said?
- Could this belief be true only because you've said it to yourself too many times?
- Are you confusing a belief with a bad habit?
- Is your thought loaded with all-or-nothing terms, exaggerated phrases, or other terminology that is part of distorted thinking?
- Are you overgeneralizing the event?

Here's an example of how it works:

1. ASK YOURSELF:

What was the thought? I look disgusting in a swimsuit.

Translate what this thought is telling me. I'm never going to be happy with my body.

How does this thought make me feel? Embarrassed at the way I look and disgusted that I don't do something about it.

How much do I believe this thought on a scale of 1 to 10, with 10 being the most? 10

If I didn't think this way, how could I look at the situation differently? I wouldn't feel so intimidated at the beach.

2. LOOK FOR THE EVIDENCE:

Is there any truth to this thought? Yes, I know what I see in the mirror.

State the evidence to support my thought. Who said you look terrible in a swimsuit? Nobody says it to me. I just know it's true.

State the evidence against it. Well, my boyfriend is always telling me to take off my cover-up. He tells me all the time that I'm beautiful.

How would someone neutral view this situation? Nobody on the beach has a perfect body.

3. MODIFY THE THOUGHT:

What's a more rational way for me to look at the situation? This is who I am and how I look. I can love myself for who I am now, even though I desire to change.

What would I tell someone else in the same situation? Practically nobody thinks they look great in a swimsuit.

What should I be telling myself? I accept myself as I am.

Now it's your turn. Go through this exercise with the emotions and automatic thoughts you uncovered in Step 3. Every time you feel the same negative voice in your head, come back to this exercise. Always keep in mind that your emotions are dominated by thoughts, however unconscious they may be. There is space for you to practice below, or you can download the exercise called "Automatic Thoughts Challenge" on my Web site, www.elizakingsford.com.

1. ASK YOURSELF:

What was the thought?

_____

_____

_____

Translate what this thought is telling me:

_____

_____

_____

How does this thought make me feel?

_____

_____

_____

How much do I believe this thought on a scale of 1 to 10, with 10
being the most? _____

If I didn't think this way, how could I look at the situation differently?

_____

_____

_____

2. LOOK FOR THE EVIDENCE:

Is there any truth to this thought?

_____

_____

_____

State the evidence to support my thought:

_____

_____

_____

State the evidence against it:

_____

_____

_____

How would someone neutral view this situation?

_____

_____

_____

3. MODIFY THE THOUGHT:

What's a more rational way for me to look at the situation?

_____

_____

_____

What would I tell someone else in the same situation?

_____

_____

_____

What should I be telling myself?

_____

_____

_____

UN-PREDICTING THE FUTURE

Another way our automatic thoughts work against us is through the cognitive distortion I described in Step 3 called fortune-telling. We do this a lot in our personal lives. For example, breaking off a relationship can make us "predict" that we'll never be happy again. Believing we're overweight can make us "predict" we'll never get married. Thinking we're not smart enough can make us "predict" we'll never get into graduate school, so we don't even try. All of these things, like so many life events, can unconsciously make us find solace in food.

When we engage in fortune-telling, it is easy to turn what we fear will happen into a self-fulfilling prophecy, especially when it comes to weight loss. The end goal seems so far away, we predict that it will never happen—and it _doesn't_ happen, because we feel disillusioned and give up. For example, a traveling salesman might predict, "I'm on the road all the time, and there's no way I can eat healthy." An upcoming cruise might make you predict, "There is no way I am NOT going to gain A LOT of weight on this vacation." Getting back in the workforce might make you predict, "I'll never find time to get any exercise." They can all make you conclude, "The cards are stacked against me. What's the use in trying?"

We're all guilty of making negative predictions from time to time, but is it habitual in your life? Has fortune-telling caused interference in your past plans to lose weight, exercise, and adopt a healthy lifestyle? Making negative predictions is another way we insinuate "I can'ts" into our lives. Most often, negative predictions turn into reality because we subconsciously make it a foregone conclusion and then act accordingly. During your weight-loss journey, you undoubtedly will do some fortune-telling, which is why the following exercise is an important Dealing Skill. It's one I predict will serve you well to use a lot. Using the previous examples, here's how to go about it.

Identifying Negative Predictions

1. **My negative prediction:** I travel too much for work, so trying to eat healthy all the time is impossible.

    How I make this prediction come true: Since I can't control what's on my plate and I'm forced to eat out so much, I just order what looks good. What's the use, since I don't know what's in it?

    Ways to disprove the prediction: I know where I am going to be each day, so I can research where I can eat, look up the menus online, and, the night before, select what I will eat the next day. I will always carry healthy snacks with me so I never get caught in a situation where I am so hungry and have to eat on the fly. I will choose to do my best each day.

2. **My negative prediction:** I am going on a cruise—not my idea!—and I know there is no way I am *not* going to gain *a lot* of weight. Everyone does.

    How I make this prediction come true: A cruise is all about eating, so food will be tempting me all day. I'm sure I'll end up eating whatever I want whenever I feel like it just because "it's there," even if I'm not hungry.

    Ways to disprove the prediction: Tracking my food intake on this trip is super important, and I will do it every day. With all the food that is served, there will always be plenty of healthy choices, if I take the time to look for them. I will survey the buffet table first, then decide what to eat, then take a seat far away from the buffet. Also, I will make sure to hit the ship's gym every morning.

3.   **My negative prediction:** I'm going back to work now that my kids are in school. It's a desk job and I still have a busy home life, so I know there will be no time for the gym.

   How I make this prediction come true: If I don't plan to exercise each day, most likely it won't happen.

   Ways to disprove the prediction: I'll commit to hitting the gym every day at lunch by making it a daily goal. (You'll learn all about goal setting in Step 8.) Even better, I'll sign up for a spinning class and put it in my daily schedule. If I can't get to the gym at lunch, certainly I can take a walk.

Think of the reservations you may have right now about losing weight, getting more movement into your life, and adopting a healthy lifestyle. Now call them what they are—negative predictions—and deny them with the following exercise. You can do the exercise here or download the worksheet called "Negative Prediction Skill" from my Web site, www.elizakingsford.com.

What Would My Best Friend Say?

You and your best friend are getting dressed to go out on the town. You look at her in her minidress and form-fitting sweater, then look in the mirror at yourself in your tights and long sweater to cover up your bulges. You feel fat and not so attractive, and blurt out, "Go without me. I can't find anything decent to wear. I look bad in everything."

Really? *Really?* Is that what your best friend is thinking, too? Of course not! She'd probably say, "That outfit looks great on you." And it probably does. You may not be able to wear her outfit, but the one you're in is attractive on you.

Our cognitive distortions do just that—give us a distorted image of ourselves, one that is never flattering and is often self-defeating. Every time you feel down in the dumps over what you're thinking or feeling, seek the real truth by asking yourself, "What would my best friend say?" This is the person who sees the best in you—always. By the same token, you must always shake off your negative thoughts and see the best in yourself.

1. My negative prediction:

    _____

    _____

    _____

    How I make this prediction come true:

    _____

    _____

    _____

    Ways to disprove the prediction:

    _____

    _____

    _____

2. My negative prediction:

    _____

    _____

    _____

    How I make this prediction come true:

    _____

    _____

    _____

    Ways to disprove the prediction:

    _____

    _____

    _____

3. My negative prediction:

    _____

    _____

    _____

How I make this prediction come true:

_____

_____

_____

Ways to disprove the prediction:

_____

_____

_____

When it comes to negative fortune-telling, this is the time you want to prove yourself wrong! Do it every opportunity you get.

FINDING YOUR WISE MIND

As I explained in Step 4, your Wise Mind is the synthesis of your emotional and reasonable minds—when your reason is informed by your emotions and your emotions are informed by your reason. Consider your Wise Mind like your North Star. It knows how to guide your thoughts when they start to stray. To help you recognize your cognitive distortions and abort their mission, practice this exercise.

To get started, go back to Step 3 where you identified the cognitive distortions that are driving your mind-set. Your cognitive distortions will be your practice tools. Follow through as to how the distortion typically unfolds and how you can insert your Wise Mind to bring on a positive outcome. Here is an example of how it works.

Cognitive Distortion(s): Labeling and Mislabeling

Describe the situation that put you in this mind-set: I went out for breakfast and ordered the flight of pancakes with a side of bacon instead of the veggie omelet I had planned. And I ate every last bite— butter, syrup, and all.

What was your automatic thought? I have no self-control. I'm such a loser.

What emotion(s) were you feeling? Disgust with myself and failure.

Where would you place your emotion(s) on a scale of 1 to 10, with 1 being the worst? 2

What behavior is your feeling creating? When I screw up like this, I find it impossible to get back on plan and I end up eating poorly for the rest of the day.

What would be the automatic thought of a wiser mind? Oops, I ordered the wrong thing, but it's only one meal and the first of the day. Get right back on track starting now, and I won't ruin anything.

What would be the emotion of a wiser mind? Determination

Where would this emotion fit on a scale of 1 to 10, with 10 being most exuberant? 8

What would be the behavior of a wiser mind? Track the over-the-top breakfast just the same as any other day and make smart food decisions for the rest of the day.

This is the ideal scenario, but it is acted out on paper. If this were acted out in real life, perhaps the best your Wise Mind could emote is disappointment, which would fit on the scale at about a 5. That's okay because it's better—you didn't fall victim to a self-defeating mind-set. Becoming the master of your own mind takes practice. Every time you feel yourself being overcome by a cognitive distortion, go through this practice. You can start here, or go to my Web site, www.elizakingsford.com, and download the worksheet "Cognitive Distortions Challenge."

Cognitive Distortion(s):

_____

_____

_____

Describe the situation that put you in this mind-set:

_____

_____

_____

What was your automatic thought?

_____

_____

_____

What emotion(s) were you feeling?

_____

_____

_____

Where would you place your emotion(s) on a scale of 1 to 10, with 1 being the worst?

_____

_____

_____

What behavior is your feeling creating?

_____

_____

_____

What would be the automatic thought of a wiser mind?

_____

_____

_____

What would be the emotion of a wiser mind?

_____

_____

_____

Where would this emotion fit on a scale of 1 to 10, with 10 being most exuberant?

_____

_____

_____

What would be the behavior of a wiser mind?

_____

_____

_____

SHORE UP YOUR SUPPORT SYSTEM

You've lost and gained and lost and gained so often, you're feeling you just can't tell anybody you're trying to do it again. You feel your spouse will only roll his eyes and mutter, "How long is it going to last this time?" Or maybe the wound is still raw from the time your son rebuked a compliment on your weight loss with, "Give her a month and she'll gain it all back."

Past failures often mean that the next try will be endeavored without telling anybody. That only makes the work harder, the journey lonelier, and the risk of another failure greater. This time, though, is different because this time you are *not going on another diet*. This time, you are adopting a healthy lifestyle, one that has no end but is a continuous journey in healthy living—and that's different because it's empowering! Every little step is an achievement toward success, toward your own Healthy Obsession. Your Dealing Skills are

BITS Lead to Overeating

Overeating doesn't just "happen." There is *always* some emotion or situation that precipitates the urge to eat "because I feel like it." When your mind starts moving you in this direction, stop, pause, take a slow, deep breath, and ask yourself:

- Am I **B**ored?

- Am I **I**rritated?

- Am I **T**ired?

- Am I **S**tressed?

These are BITS, the four most common situations that cause us to make decisions we are not happy with—such as going on an all-out binge. You are definitely not thinking with your Wise Mind when you are in any of these moods.

If you find yourself with an urge to overeat or eat when you're not hungry, pause and question your BITS. If you answer yes to any one of them, use one of your best-working Dealing Skills to pull your mind in another direction.

in place to help make it happen. Keep in mind, however, that many of the behaviors and thoughts you've been working to correct have an antecedent, often other people. They can be a powerful force: "Let's order this." "Forget the gym." "Have another beer." "Don't be such a straight arrow." And you hate to disappoint.

In the ideal world, your quest for Healthy Obsession would be embraced by your immediate family (possibly), your most intimate circle of friends (hopefully), and other people who you interact with in your daily or almost daily life (maybe). In reality, though, at best one or two people, but possibly no one, will be joining you. Whatever path the people in your world choose to follow, you will serve yourself best by firmly and confidently letting them *all* know, "I am on the path to a healthy lifestyle and I need your help." In return, you should be able to depend on some, if not all, of those in your innermost circle of importance to support you in your mission.

Resolve Conflict without Confrontation

Being in conflict with someone is risky business because it heightens emotions that can drive you to food. Many people are constantly living in conflict with certain people in their lives who they can't avoid—a co-worker, a spouse who couldn't care less about their healthy pursuit, or an in-law who is always needling them about their weight. You'll best serve yourself by getting this emotional baggage out of your life. Here's how to do it without damaging a relationship.

1. Describe the situation to the person you are in conflict with in a nonjudgmental way: "Sweetheart, I really don't want you to keep bringing home ice cream."

2. Tell the person how the situation makes you feel: "When you bring ice cream into the house, I feel like you don't care that I am trying to change my eating habits."

3. Be mindful by avoiding blame words and exhibiting intense emotion. Say, "I would love and appreciate if you'd support me," not, "You're the reason I can't lose weight!"

4. Tell the person exactly what you need and would like them to do: "Please buy only the items on the shopping list and nothing more."

A small army of supporters can actually be a mighty fortress protecting your best interests. Just knowing they are there will mentally help you stay accountable to your goals. You should be able to count on your supporters to encourage you in your moments of weakness when cognitive distortions turn up the volume in your head, when difficult triggers cross your path, and when stressful situations start to fray at your resolve.

Who in your inner circle will have your back when other people or circumstances challenge you? Who in your inner circle are the ones who might be the challengers and be more difficult to rein in? "Come on, let's go get some pizza," or "You don't have time for the gym today, you have family obligations, you know," or "You've worked really hard losing all that weight. You *deserve* to eat big tonight." Other people you routinely interact with might be a challenge. It's important for you to know how your world of interpersonal relationships stacks up.

Prepare yourself by making a list of all your closest friends, relatives, acquaintances, and co-workers who you routinely interact with or socialize with and think about how they might respond to your new and improved life. For example, I had one client who was part of an "in-crowd" clique of co-workers who always sat at the same lunch table every day. When Ellen announced she was "changing her eating habits" and asked for her friends' support, she got a unified affirmative from all of them. However, the person she considered "my best friend at work" was always trying to bait her. "Carol is always stopping by my office to ask 'How is it going?' with a doughnut or bagel or some other food in her hand. She clearly did not like what I was doing. She's a little overweight, too, and I think she feels threatened that I'm doing something about it and she's not." Turned out Ellen was right. To get away from Carol, she started packing her own lunch and eating in her office. Ellen wound up putting an end to their friendship because she decided the relationship wasn't serving her. If her "best friend" didn't really want her to be healthier and happier, she wasn't really a "best friend" now, was she?

Quite often people themselves are triggers. My client Nick stuck to his goals just fine except for the times when his old pal Eric showed up in his life. Eric would egg Nick on to go out drinking and stay out too late, which sent Nick so off plan it would take him several days to recover. Eric was a trigger that Nick subdued by texting NOT GOING! instead of answering the call and listening to Eric plead until he gave in.

Are there any Carols and Nicks in your life? On the flip side, who are the people you know who will be your biggest backers? What role will the people who are routinely in your life play in your health quest—good, bad, or otherwise? You need to know so you can be prepared. Download the document "My Support Group" from my Web site, www.elizakingsford.com, for your notebook, or do this exercise in your journal or the space provided. Here is an example of what it might look like.

Person	Relationship	Role in My Health Quest
Jim	Spouse	Supported me in the past, but after too many failures may doubt my intentions this time.
Betsy	Neighbor who I go to happy hour with every Wednesday.	Probably won't be happy to hear that I want to break this habit. Get ready to be firm about my new lifestyle.
Nancy	My BFF	She'll be thrilled and most likely be my biggest supporter.
Liz	Sister	She's been on me to get serious about weight loss for years. A definite supporter.

Now it's your turn.

Person	Relationship	Role in My Health Quest

My support group will be:

1. _____

2. _____

3. _____

4. _____

5. _____

You have two obligations to your supporters in exchange for their help. You need to be assertive about your needs and not be timid about asking for help when you need it. They need to feel you are confident and determined. Here's how to go about it:

Be clear about your intentions. Communicate and clarify. For example, tell your husband, "I am committed to my healthy lifestyle, so I need to clear the house of the goldfish crackers right now. I don't want that temptation in the house."

Speak with positive affirmation. For example, tell your family, "We are eating vegetables at every meal because we are pursuing health," not "We are all eating vegetables at every meal, so don't argue with me." Always ask yourself, "How would I respond if I was spoken to that way?"

Lead with your Wise Mind. Be patient and mindful of those around you, especially when making requests. Speak with your Wise Mind: "I know vegetables aren't your favorite, but we are a healthy family and eating vegetables is part of that. I'd like you to at least try them and decide if you hate them as much as you say you do." Never speak with your Emotional Mind: "You'll eat what's on your plate and that's that. I don't care if you like them or not."

Assert your needs. Be assertive when you need your voice to be heard in a group: "I'd like to order something other than pizza for lunch. Who all is with me?" Once someone goes against an assumed majority, others usually follow suit.

State your thoughts carefully. Use "I statements" and not "blame statements": "I'm really focused on my health right now, so I'm going to choose to stay in tonight," not "She serves nothing but junk at her parties. I wouldn't be caught dead there."

Be firm about your needs. Do not apologize or demean yourself when making a request. Phrases like "I hate to ask" or "I'm such a pest, do you mind if . . ." do not serve you because people may not take you seriously.

As I told you from the start, moving your mind-set away from cognitive distortions and getting your emotions in check takes practice, practice, practice. As you do so, your wise mind will gradually start taking hold. But where is it all leading? What is the healthy lifestyle and the healthy eating I've been referring to all about? It's now time you found out.

MASTER OF WEIGHT LOSS: Eileen M.

"My Problem Was More about Me Than It Was about Food"

I'd been battling my weight for as long as I could remember—at least 30 years. I got to the point where I was just so tired of thinking about my struggle with food, exercise, and my body. No matter what diet or exercise program I tried, nothing worked. I couldn't lose weight and keep it off, and I couldn't just be happy where I was. I felt stuck and hopeless. I found Eliza Kingsford because I decided it was time to look for answers that ran deeper than my diet.

I have to admit I was skeptical at first about seeing a psychotherapist about my diet, even though I knew she specialized in weight loss. She asked me about my family history (who else in my family was overweight) and what my eating habits and exercise habits were. We made some small dietary changes to get me started, and then we got into what I believe was the heart of things. She started asking me about how I talk to myself and my body. I thought she was nuts at first. How I talk to my body? What does that even mean? She had me do some exercises she called Dealing Skills, which got me to realize that I was sending myself a consistent stream of negative messages every day, and I wasn't really even aware of it. I was starting to see that my problem was more about me than it was about food.

My day looked something like this: Wake up and look in the mirror to brush my teeth and say something mean about how my face or hair looked. As I got dressed, I'd berate my body in front of the mirror while I put my clothes on. By then, I was not feeling great about myself, and I'd trudge into the kitchen. Perhaps I'd be a little short with my husband, who'd respond by snapping at me. I'd wallow in my food decisions for the morning, finally feeling exasperated and reaching for something that would soothe me. This only made me more frustrated with myself because I'd made the wrong food choice—again.

Together, Eliza and I started identifying my automatic thoughts and negative assumptions about myself, and how they would lead to messages and behaviors that I wasn't happy with. Slowly, she asked me to start replacing those messages with ones that were more self-compassionate and kind. She told me that once I started taking care of myself and my mind, I would be more inclined to take care of my body and more determined about what I put in my mouth. I practiced deflecting my negative messages until I was no longer getting bogged down by negative self-talk. Not only was I more willing to choose food and movement behaviors that were working in my favor, but I was also able to cut myself some slack about my shape and my weight. Strangely enough, when I started to get good at this, my weight came off naturally. Slow but steady. I learned how to have compassion and love for myself while I was working on getting healthier and changing my shape. I felt more at peace with my body and with my mind. I am still a work in progress, but I feel so much happier than I did when I was fighting my body and dieting like crazy.

Adopt a New Lifestyle of Healthy Eating

H ere's the question you've likely been pondering since you read Step 1: How do you lose weight and keep it off without going on a diet? The answer is the reality that all Long-Term Weight Controllers (LTWCs) come to embrace: You do it by making the commitment to trade in your current food habits in favor of a healthy style of eating.

And how do you do that? By courting a brand-new relationship with food, which kicks off by affirming, "I am done with dieting. I am just going to eat what's best for me nutritionally." And that brings me to Brain-Powered Pointer No. 11:

> Food in your body is like gasoline in your car:
> Quality enhances performance.

It's foolhardy for me or anyone else to dictate what and how much of something you can and should eat in order to lose weight. It simply is impossible to accurately predict, within a reasonable margin of error, an individual's caloric and nutritional needs. And if anybody tries to tell you that they can, they are only deluding you. One-size-fits-all diets and programs that prescribe calories and/or fat, protein, and carbohydrate ratios don't work over the long haul because they can't take into account everybody's unique metabolism and how it reacts to the macronutrients (protein, fat, and carbs) and micronutrients (vitamins, minerals, and phytonutrients) in the foods you eat. The only way to do this accurately would be to hook you up to a machine each day that takes into account all the factors that affect your metabolism and spits out how many calories you burned—hardly practical! As I noted in Step 2, it's why two people identical in age, height, and weight who eat exactly the same thing over a specific time frame will not lose the same amount of weight. They'll also gain it back at a different pace.

For this reason, I am not going to lay out a day-to-day diet for you, dictate how many calories you must eat, and offer menu plans. This only perpetuates the notion that "dieting" is a means with a so-called end. Besides, if I did, you'd only get bored in due time, just like you did following diets in the past. Rather, I am going to show you how to design your own plan within your personal caloric requirements by making the optimal choices that will nourish and satisfy you. Over time, your new healthy eating effort will turn into a new stick-with-it habit, one that will get you well on your way to Healthy Obsession. It's a style of eating you're going to love because you'll be eating foods you love—or are learning to love. You're also going to love it because you're going to look and feel better, and, this I can promise, you're going to get to a healthy weight for your body.

Instead of a "diet," I offer you 10 Principles of Healthy Eating designed to drive your food decisions in terms of quality and nutrition. They are simple to follow, sustainable over the long haul, and based on scientific findings as to what dietary practices are best in terms of weight loss, long-term success, and overall good health. You are free to make your own healthy food choices based on these principles. In fact, I want you to get comfortable making your own food choices without having to depend on a so-called diet or diet recipes.

You may be familiar with some of these principles; others, or maybe all, may be new to you. Perhaps you are already adhering to some of them. Whatever your nutritional circumstance is at the moment, do not feel that you have to adopt all 10 principles at once. The only thing you must do to get started is to adopt Principle 1 (the heart of healthy eating) and Principle 2 (your accountability system). You can enlist the other eight one at a time or according to your own comfort level. Studies show that gradually adopting healthy eating habits will lead to sustainable weight loss. In these studies, people who successfully achieved weight loss did not try to change everything at once. They mastered one new skill, then layered on another, then another. I encourage you to do the same.

Look at these 10 principles and think about which ones are most realistic to incorporate into your life right now and which ones you can put off until your new eating style starts taking hold. However, you must aim to eventually adopt them all. Putting them all into practice is the way you'll see the results you want and is the only way you'll maintain your weight loss. When it comes to food choices, these 10 principles are what having a Healthy Obsession is all about.

If you stick to these nutritional principles as best you can, you *will* lose weight—naturally and gradually—without the burden of "being on a diet." Doing so will be easier than ever before because you are simultaneously getting the mental fortitude to make it happen by practicing the exercises in this book. Combining sound nutrition with the mental resilience practices you are learning is your best chance to make weight loss permanent and become an LTWC yourself! Even if it's a struggle at first, just keep at it, which brings me to Brain-Powered Pointer No. 12:

> Consistency over time will lead to making this
> style of eating your new lifelong habit.

Before we get to the principles, I want to help you understand why weight loss is such a struggle and will continue to get harder if you don't change your relationship with food. Consider it more must-have knowledge that will help bolster your resolve. The reason you are overweight is not your fault.

As I explained in the Introduction, there are many forces working against our best intentions to eat healthier and lose weight. Our exposure to too much of the wrong kinds of foods practically 24/7 is a major one. The marketing messages designed to make highly caloric and high-fat foods sound like the only kinds of food we should be eating is another. Then there is a problem that scientists only in the past few years have started to explore—our propensity to become addicted to certain foods.

THE PROBLEM OF FOOD ADDICTION

There is emerging scientific proof that many of us can get hooked on eating in the same way people get addicted to cigarettes and illicit drugs. It's not happening with good-for-you natural foods such as spinach and oatmeal. The foods that can trigger an addictive response are processed items such as pizza, french fries, chocolate, chips, and ice cream—foods that are intentionally enhanced with refined sugar and/or fat for greater taste appeal and appetite satisfaction.

Breakthrough human studies published in the medical journal *PLOS One* found that people who eat certain processed foods share common behavioral patterns with other addictive disorders by releasing dopamine, what is known as the feel-good hormone. And just as with heroin, cocaine, and cigarettes, it gradually requires more indulging to elicit a dopamine response. More than 90 percent of the people in the study who identified as a food addict reported a "persistent desire or repeated unsuccessful attempt to quit."

"Addictive substances are rarely in their natural state, but have been altered or processed in a manner that increases their abuse potential," the study reported. "For example, grapes are processed into wine and poppies are refined into opium. A similar process may be occurring within our food supply."

Researchers noted that there are natural foods that contain sugar (such as fruit) and fat (such as nuts), but sugar and fat rarely occur naturally in the same food. Many highly palatable foods, such as pizza, chocolate, and cake, have been processed to have artificially elevated levels of both. "In our modern food environment, there has been a steep increase in the availability of what is referred to as 'highly processed foods,'" the researchers wrote. "It is plausible that like drugs of abuse, these highly processed foods may be more likely to trigger addictive-like biological and behavioral responses due to their . . . high levels of reward."

The conveyance of the reward system has been linked to the way highly processed foods induce a blood sugar spike. "This is important because there is a known link between glucose levels and activation of areas of the brain that are involved in addiction," the researchers reported.

Blood sugar rise is measured by what is known as glycemic index (GI), the speed at which glucose enters the bloodstream, and glycemic load (GL), which also accounts for the amount of carbohydrates creating the spike. The research suggests that the nature of an addictive food correlates to the potency of its glycemic load.

What all this means is that you may be struggling to resist certain foods not so much because you love the taste, but because of the way the chemicals in the food make the reward center in your brain react, causing you to overeat these foods and desire them on a consistent basis.

Are You a Food Addict?

Generally speaking, people who struggle with a food addiction are likely to be overweight or obese. However, not all people who are overweight or obese have a food addiction. Here's how you can find out where you stand.

Read through this list of common addictive foods and check off those you either have a tendency to overeat or have a hard time stopping once you start eating them. Then answer the questions that follow to the best of your ability. If you prefer to do this exercise in the privacy of your journal or notebook, you can download the worksheet "Are You a Food Addict?" from my Web site, www.elizakingsford.com.

☐ Bread and rolls (especially white)

☐ Burgers

☐ Cake

☐ Candy

☐ Cereal

☐ Cheese

☐ Chips

☐ Chocolate anything

☐ Cookies

☐ Crackers

☐ Doughnuts

☐ French fries

☐ Fried chicken or other deep-fried protein

☐ Ice cream

☐ Muffins

☐ Pasta

☐ Pizza

☐ Popcorn (buttered)

☐ Salami

☐ Sausages

☐ Soft drinks (non-diet)

☐ Others not on this list:

_____

Think back to your consumption of any of these foods over the last year and answer the following questions.

During the Past Year

	Never (0)	Almost Never (1)	Sometimes (2)	Almost Always (3)	Always (4)
1. When I eat this food(s), I end up eating more than I planned to.					
2. I find myself eating this food(s) even when I'm not hungry.					
3. I often feel sluggish or fatigued after overeating.					
4. I often eat to the point where I feel sick.					
5. I find myself snacking on this food(s) throughout the day.					
6. When I am hungry for this food and it's not in the house, I will go out of my way to get it.					
7. I have a tendency to want to eat this food(s) when I'm feeling emotional, such as when I'm angry, happy, worried, anxious, or moody.					

(continued)

During the Past Year *(cont.)*

	Never (0)	Almost Never (1)	Sometimes (2)	Almost Always (3)	Always (4)
8. I struggle with trying to cut down or stop eating this food(s).					
9. Sometimes, I prefer to eat this food(s) instead of working, spending time with family or friends, or engaging in physical activities or personal interests.					
10. When I overeat this food(s), I am consumed with guilt or other negative emotions.					
11. There are times when I avoid situations (parties, activities, etc.) because I am worried I will overeat.					
12. There are times when I avoid social situations because I know I will be in the presence of certain food(s).					

	Never (0)	Almost Never (1)	Sometimes (2)	Almost Always (3)	Always (4)
13. Overeating this food(s) and/or overeating in general causes me to wallow in cognitive distortions.					
14. When I try to cut this food(s) out of my diet, I experience symptoms of withdrawal, such as agitation and anxiety.					
15. Fasting from this food(s) increases my desire for it (them) after a few days.					
16. Eating this food(s) and/or overeating in general interferes with my home, family, and/or personal life.					
17. I have unsuccessfully tried to avoid eating this food(s) or stop overeating in general.					

(continued)

During the Past Year *(cont.)*

	Never (0)	Almost Never (1)	Sometimes (2)	Almost Always (3)	Always (4)
18. Over time I have found that I need to eat more and more to get the feeling I want, such as increasing pleasure or reducing a negative emotion.					
19. My overweight has caused significant psychological problems, such as depression, anxiety, guilt, or self-loathing.					
20. My overweight has led to other weight-related health problems.					

Based on the Yale Food Addiction Scale by Ashley N. Gearhardt, PhD; William R. Corbin, PhD; and Kelly D. Brownell, PhD (2009).

Scoring

Add up your total score to the 20 questions. Here is what the results are telling you.

0–20	You don't appear to have a food addiction, but may have a tendency to overeat the wrong foods.
21–40	You might struggle trying to avoid certain foods because of their addictive nature, and you are successful only part of the time.

| 41–60 | You might have a food addiction that could be interfering with your ability to lose weight and/or keep it off. |
| 61–80 | You might have a food addiction that could be causing you considerable personal distress. |

Keep in mind that just because you may not fit the profile for having a food addiction does not mean that you don't have a negative reaction to certain foods. Addiction specialist Brad Lamm calls it being "addicted, afflicted, or affected." If you have a food habit that you find hard to break, it's likely you fall into one of these three categories. And the more you eat the foods that are affecting you in that way, the more you'll want to eat them. The way to wean yourself away from these foods is to replace them with healthy foods. Just like with an addiction to cigarettes, studies show that the longer you stay away from foods that do not serve you, the less interested you will be in them over time. In other words, the same 10 Principles of Healthy Eating that lead to sustained weight loss are also designed to help break the food habits of those who are addicted, afflicted, or affected.

THE 10 PRINCIPLES OF HEALTHY EATING

The food component of Brain-Powered Weight Loss is a habit-forming lifestyle change that emphasizes nutrient-dense whole foods and discourages processed, overly fatty, and sugar-laden choices. All the principles are backed by research showing that each of them benefits health and can naturally take off pounds. This is a simple-to-follow approach that does not bog you down with a lot of rules. Each of the 10 principles works synergistically, so adopting one makes it easier to practice the next and the next. Remember, you can adopt them at your own speed, but success is contingent on adopting them all.

Research shows that adherence to adopting a healthier lifestyle is highly variable. Success is dose dependent, meaning positive results are associated with more frequent and consistent healthy choices. The more you embrace these principles and actively follow them, the faster you will reach your desired outcome. There are plenty of full-of-flavor options for what you can eat. The choice is all yours. When you switch to the 10 Principles of Healthy Eating, the only thing left starving are your fat cells!

Principle No. 1: Focus on Nutrient-Dense Whole Foods

In other words, eat foods in their purist form, or as close to it as possible, with no-to-minimal processing whenever you can. This means foods taken straight from their natural state and sold to you that way, without additives, artificial coloring, and/or processing. Replacing processed foods with nutrient-dense whole food choices is the prime driver for ending food addiction and reaching your optimal healthy weight.

Eating whole foods means being mindful of desiring a healthy relationship with food. It's about choosing fresh foods from the farmers' market or supermarket instead of eating out of a box or bag. It's about avoiding refined (white) starches and added sugars as best you can. It's about planning a meal around proteins you find in the fresh meat or fish department instead of pre-packaged meals from the frozen foods compartment, even if they are marketed as a "diet meal." It's about eating out less and cooking more so you are in control of what you put in your body. Overall, it's about valuing nutrition more than convenience.

Choosing natural whole foods as an alternative to convenience is important because processed foods compromise nutrition and work against your efforts to lose weight. Processing often removes or reduces the nutrients in whole foods that are naturally rich in vitamins, minerals, and fiber and replaces them with excessive amounts of fat, sugar, and sodium. Processed foods typically contain artificial flavorings and coloring to make them more palatable. The additives and preservatives necessary to give them shelf life work against you because they are not natural. Eating foreign substances confuses your body because it doesn't recognize them as energy and doesn't know what to do with them, so it converts them to fat and stores it. If it doesn't get burned as fuel, it adds up to unwanted extra pounds. It is no coincidence that the popularity of packaged foods and fast-food establishments in this country parallels our rising obesity epidemic!

Eating nutrient-dense whole foods puts the emphasis on fresh fruits and vegetables, whole grains that have not been bleached or enriched, and proteins such as chicken, fish, seafood, and limited amounts of lean red meat. A nutrient-dense whole food regimen also includes healthier fats (Principle No. 6), found in certain oils and foods such as salmon, walnuts, and flaxseeds. There is no

Defining "Processed"

Not all convenience foods are created equal. Some items do you no nutritional harm, such as frozen fruits and vegetables, unsalted canned beans and vegetables, many dairy products, whole grains, nut butters, and unsalted organic broths and stock. Here's how to tell when an item does do you harm: Check the list of ingredients. If it contains ingredients that you can't find in a grocery store and that sound like they came out of a chemistry lab, consider the food processed. The longer the list, the greater the processing.

place for artificial anything on a whole foods regimen, especially trans fats and artificial sweeteners.

Eating nutritiously dense whole foods makes good weight-loss sense because they naturally increase satiety. This is due, in part, to the effect of the natural fiber and water found in all fruits and vegetables; the high protein content of lean meats, poultry, and fish; and the good heart-healthy fats found in avocado, coconut, olive, and nut oils. When you look at the ideal whole foods plate, it looks like this:

- One-half fruits and vegetables, with the emphasis on the veggies
- One-quarter whole grains, minimally processed
- One-quarter protein—fish, seafood, poultry, lean game or meat

The kinds of foods you will find on the plate include:

- All fresh fruits
- All fresh vegetables
- Dairy (sparingly)
- Eggs
- Fish
- Lean meat
- Lean skinless poultry and game
- Legumes

- Nuts

- Oils, such as olive, coconut, avocado, and nut

- Whole grains

Principle No. 2: Self-Monitor with Scrutiny

Here's a challenge for you: Name everything you ate yesterday. How about everything you put in your mouth the day before or last Tuesday? Do you know how many calories or how much sugar you eat day to day? Impossible to say, right? Not if you keep track of what you're eating every day, which brings me to Brain-Powered Pointer No. 13:

You can't manage what you don't monitor.

Study after study has found that the single most important tactic people use to achieve successful and sustained weight loss is to track their food and calorie intake in a food diary. And this research was conducted before the advent of apps and smartphones, when you had to find calorie counts by looking them up in a book and adding everything up manually! Now it is easier than ever because your smartphone does all the work. Just download any number of free apps, follow the instructions, and you're on your way.

For example, I use and recommend to clients the free app at myfitnesspal .com. Setting it up and getting started is easy. You punch in personal data, and it will give you an approximate number of calories to eat, based on the goals you set for yourself in the system. I say "approximate," because it can't account for your metabolism and the other metabolic factors I discussed in Step 2, so consider this number only as a guideline. Then, you're ready to go. All you need to do is enter what you eat and, in an instant, it will give you the calories plus an entire range of important (and not-so-important) nutritional data.

The app has thousands of name brands and dishes in its database, plus information from all the restaurant chains, including regional ones, that post nutritional data. Let's say you're persuaded to stop at a local Italian restaurant where you know nothing about the menu and the owner doesn't have to disclose the nutritional value of his dishes. Interested in eggplant parm? In an instant, your app will give you a generic value of the dish. Love your own homemade eggplant parm? Just enter your recipe ingredients, and it will give you all the nutritional data and store it for you, so next time you eat it, it's a one-click entry. In addition, the app will also store the data of all the sand-wiches, soups, and other dishes you eat on a regular basis.

Let's look at its usefulness another way. Let's say you think you don't eat enough fiber (Principle No. 7), so you set a goal to eat 30 grams a day. Track it and see how close you are. You might be surprised to find out how little fiber you were eating before. Same goes for calories, fat, carbohydrates, or whatever other nutritional value is of interest to you.

Try tracking your food intake for a few days *before* you start adjusting your diet. It will give you good insight into how many calories you've typically been eating day to day. Clients often tell me that they had no idea how much they

Breakfast and Weight-Loss Champions

Results from scientific studies are mixed on whether skipping break-fast helps or hurts weight-loss efforts, but here's what we know about Long-Term Weight Controllers: Eating something in the morning is a definite benefit.

Nearly 80 percent of people who have lost 30 pounds or more and kept it off for at least a year say they eat breakfast daily, accord-ing to data from the National Weight Control Registry, which tracks the dietary and behavioral habits of more than 10,000 successful losers. The reason: Eating helps wake up your metabolism, research shows. Studies also show that people who eat breakfast are more focused and are better able to maintain a healthy weight.

A lot of people skip breakfast as a way to save calories for later in the day, which is risky thinking, because it can so easily backfire. You can end up famished a few hours into the day and reach for anything you can swallow fast, or compensate by overeating at lunch or dinner. One study found that breakfast eaters actually consume about 7 per-cent fewer calories throughout the day and overall eat a healthier diet than breakfast skippers.

If food is the last thing you want when you awaken, keep in mind that it needn't be eaten before you walk out the door in the morning. Studies show that eating within 2 hours of getting up will get your metabolism in gear. So take a nutrient-dense whole food item with you, and eat it as soon as your body tells you it's ready for food.

were overeating. When you monitor, you not only keep track of what you eat, you also become aware of the quality of the food you eat. It allows you to easily make adjustments and set goals accordingly.

Other apps work in a similar way and include Lose It!, MyPlate Calorie Tracker, My Diet Coach, and Calorie Counter PRO (only for the iPhone). Most apps are interactive, so you can team up or compete with like-minded buddies. What's best is all a matter of personal preference. Whatever you choose, I recommend you do your tracking on your smartphone rather than your computer, because your phone is handy and you almost always have it with you. This is important because you should monitor what you eat as soon as you eat it, not at the end of the day. It's too easy to forget that hand-ful of peanuts you shelled and ate while perusing the menu at the corner tavern.

I'm not saying you need to monitor your food intake forever, but you should stay with it until you can assuredly mentally gauge your daily intake.

I cannot stress enough the importance of self-monitoring your food intake. It is the ideal disciplinary tool. The number one reason a lot of people start to regress, gain weight, and slip back into their old habits is because they stop being vigilant about tracking their food and exercise. Remember, if you have a weight problem, you likely have Resistant Biology that is always working against you. Letting your guard down can be like stepping into dangerous territory. When you get back to tracking, you get back on track.

Self-monitoring is not just about self-discipline; it's also about intentional-ity and awareness. It creates personal accountability for what you put in your body. If you are committed to recording everything you eat, you are more likely to be aware of the quality of the food you eat and less likely to eat foods that are not on your plan. Just as you can't buy a $2 million home on a $50,000-a-year salary without living beyond your means, you can't eat beyond your means without paying consequences. Self-monitoring is your tool for uncovering and understanding those means.

How can you manage what you don't monitor? How will you know where to adjust your eating behaviors if you don't have an accurate picture of what those behaviors are? Are you eating enough fat, protein, and fiber to keep you satiated? Enough carbohydrates to give you energy? Over time, you might find that you will naturally recognize your body's cues for these nutrients. However, until then, it's best to track your food to better understand your nutritional needs.

Principle No. 3: Be Calorie Conscious at All Times

So, exactly how many calories of wonderful natural whole foods can you eat to fulfill your wish of losing 20, 40, or possibly 100 pounds? Here's my honest answer: I have no idea.

While monitoring your calorie intake is important to losing weight, there is an inherent problem with the process. Calorie counting is an inexact science. Yes, it is partially about calories in versus calories out, and science tells us we have to burn an extra 3,500 calories to lose just 1 pound. Only it really isn't that simple; it's not the whole story. The way our bodies use calories is complex, due to our unique metabolisms. As you already learned in Step 2, we all burn calories at a different metabolic rate depending on our gender, age, height, current weight, stress level, hormone balance, and activity level. This is why your metabolic rate is not a constant. It can go up or down, depending on any combination of these changing factors. You probably know that, too, because you've gone through many 3,500-calorie deficits and didn't see the scale budge an ounce. That's the thing about calories and Resistant Biology, which brings me to Brain-Powered Pointer No. 14:

> Eating fewer calories does not mean you'll
> lose weight faster or even at all.

When your body senses a slowdown of energy coming, it does what is necessary to keep you from starving: It resists burning calories as a way to conserve fuel and slows down your metabolism.

Here's the other reality. The quality of the food you eat is way more important than the amount, because different foods have different effects on the brain's response and fat-storage systems, your satiety level, and how efficiently the food you eat is digested and turned into fuel. For example, a 300-calorie doughnut is a lot different than 300 calories worth of fruits and nuts. One is just a sugar-surging, fat-storing calorie bomb, while the other is full of satisfying fiber and satiating healthy fats.

Add up all these variables and it makes the task of counting calories seem both perplexing and frustrating. I'd love to tell you that if you eat exactly the way I describe in these principles, you don't have to count calories. But that's too risky, at least for now. If you have been struggling with weight loss, you most likely do not have a handle on what your metabolic caloric allowance really is. You need to know this, as it is your baseline level for what your consumption should be. You need to know this number so you can lose weight and maintain it. While the old energy balance equation of calories in versus calories out is largely outdated, it still holds true that you can't eat excess calories on a regular basis and maintain weight loss.

As I already said, the only way for you to know for certain your actual metabolic rate and, therefore, your precise caloric requirement is to get medically hooked up to a lot of devices that measure your oxygen intake and outtake at rest and through various activities. This is not practical or cost effective. What is practical is finding out a comfortable caloric range that will allow you to lose weight and settle in at a healthy natural weight.

The way to start is to find out what the estimated basal metabolic rate (BMR) is for someone your age and size. Just type "basal metabolic rate calculator" into the search engine of your electronic device and any number of sites can figure it out for you instantly. You just have to fill in a few details concerning your weight, height, age, and gender. I like the one found on WebMD.com, but they all work relatively the same.

Your BMR is the rate at which you burn calories when you are at rest—that is, when you are doing nothing. This will get you in the ballpark of your minimum daily requirement. The more activity you engage in during the day, the more calories your body will need.

To know what's best for you, you'll need to experiment a little. Let's say your BMR is 1,300 calories a day. If you don't do much but sit at a desk all day and you don't get much in the way of exercise, this might be your ceiling. However, if you are active every day or have a job that has you rushing around for hours on end, then your body might require considerably more calories,

Affirm Your Biological Needs

If you feel that tracking your calories is akin to being "on a diet," change that mind-set with this affirmation:
Counting calories is not about restricting my food intake; it's about being realistic about how much fuel my body requires.

perhaps an extra 500 or 1,000. Still, this may not account for other variables in your life and biology.

So, the best you can do is to take your BMR, make an estimated guess at your activity level adjustment, set a goal, stick with it, and see how your body responds. As a rule of thumb for weight loss, a very rough BMR estimate is between 1,300 and 1,800 calories a day for women and between 1,600 and 2,100 calories a day for men. Remember, though, that this can vary considerably depending on what makes you uniquely *you*. Also, keep in mind that as you lose weight, the number of calories it takes to lose or maintain weight likely will go down.

I strongly suggest that you be patient with your calorie goal and aim to lose about a pound or two a week. Remember, this is not a diet in the traditional sense; it's a lifestyle change. It's the way you want to eat forever. How you can more easily and sanely manage your calories is covered in the principles that follow.

Principle No. 4: Kick the Sugar Habit

There are lots of reasons to avoid sugar beyond its addictive nature. Sugar, particularly added sugars such as high-fructose corn syrup, has replaced fat as public health enemy number one.

American consumption of sugar is at an all-time record. We eat sugar way out of proportion to what is good for us. This is largely due to the added sugars that are snuck into our food supply through processing. On average, we eat about 7 tablespoons of sugar a day when we should be getting about 7 teaspoons, or 112 calories worth. So, if you're someone who thinks this can't be you because you never put table sugar on *anything* you eat or in anything you drink, pay close attention because virtually all of us are eating more sugar than we think.

Sugars, both the refined (dietary) kind that sit in your canisters and those added through processing, offer no health benefits. Robert Lustig, MD, endocrinologist, researcher, and author of the bestseller *Fat Chance*, has demonstrated that sugar is toxic to our bodies in ways beyond its contribution to obesity. There is a correlation between sugar intake and diabetes and heart disease. Most recently, Dr. Lustig found a link between refined and added sugar intake and nonalcoholic fatty liver disease.

Bottom line: Sugar is harmful to your health. The only exception is naturally occurring sugars, like those found in fruit and dairy foods, which contain important vitamins, minerals, fiber, and protein that promote health and satiety. These other nutrients help break down the sugar in your body in a natural way, thwarting the negative impact that dietary or added sugars have when you consume them.

When we think of sugar, we think in terms of sweets—all the pastries, cookies, cakes, ice cream, and soft drinks we covet as a treat. But that's not the primary reason we eat way too much of it. Sugar is ubiquitous in our processed and packaged foods, and its presence is not always obvious because it doesn't have to make a food taste sweet. Sugar is found in breads, breakfast cereals, jams, peanut butter, sauces, many salad dressings, jarred pasta and tomato sauces, canned pasta, and condiments such as ketchup and barbecue sauce. And that's just a very short list.

Here are a few examples of how all this sugar gets in our food supply. One cup of chopped fresh tomatoes contains 5 grams of natural sugars, but you're getting an additional 9 grams of added sugars when you eat 1 cup of marinara sauce sold in a jar. When you make your own marinara sauce, no added sugar is required. A regular serving of natural, unprocessed oatmeal contains 0 grams of sugar, but it takes 12 grams of added sugars to manufacture one packet of instant 100-calorie maple–brown sugar oatmeal. If you're hungry

---

Liquid Calories Add Up Fast

Make water your drink of choice. According to the Centers for Disease Control and Prevention (CDC), beverages contribute more sugar, calories, and artificial sweeteners to our diets than any other single consumable.

People who prefer water over diet soft drinks, alcohol, or other beverages with their meals are the same folks who eat more fruits and vegetables, eat less fast food, shop at farmers' markets, and exercise more than the typical American, says the CDC.

Think about it: A glass of orange juice at breakfast, a skinny latte with your lunch, and two glasses of wine with dinner add up to 478 calories. That's a meal's worth of calories with not much nutrition!

again an hour or two after eating this "healthy" oatmeal, it's no wonder! That added sugar is doing nothing but turning to glucose in your bloodstream, contributing to inflammation in your body, and spiking your insulin levels, resulting in a sugar crash soon after.

Here's the perfect example of why eating nutrient-dense whole foods matters. A 6-ounce package of reduced-fat plain Greek yogurt contains 6 grams of natural sugars, but it takes 19 grams of added sugars to produce a same-size container of blueberry yogurt. If you'd instead add real fresh blueberries to the same plain yogurt, you'd be eating a total of 10 grams of all-natural sugars. That's half the sugar intake, plus you'd be getting all the antioxidants and fiber found in the blueberries. It's an obvious choice.

This sugar scourge finally hit a crescendo in the spring of 2016 when the US Food and Drug Administration, despite a lot of resistance from the sugar and packaged foods industries, ruled that food labels must reveal the amount of natural sugars *and* added sugars, effective mid-2018. To people like me and others who are trying to fight our obesity epidemic, this can't happen soon enough. Take advantage of this useful tool and read food labels before buying. Your goal should be to eat as little added sugar as possible.

In an ideal world, I would recommend that you limit your sugar intake to the naturally occurring sugars found in fruits, vegetables, and dairy products. However, sugar is so pervasive in our food supply that trying to do so would be overwhelming for most people. Instead, practice what I call harm reduction, a tactic you'll learn more about in Step 9, by consciously making an assertive effort to eat as little sugar as possible. Read labels and act accordingly. Note: Added sugars come in many different guises. These are among them:

- Agave
- Barley malt
- Beet sugar
- Brown rice syrup
- Cane juice
- Cane sugar
- Corn syrup
- Dextrose
- Fructose
- Glucose
- High-fructose corn syrup
- Maltodextrin
- Maltose
- Palm sugar
- Saccharose
- Sorghum
- Sucrose

Principle No. 5: Choose Carbs with a
Low or Moderate Glycemic Load

I cringe when I hear people say they are on a low-carbohydrate diet. Here's why: Carbohydrates play a pivotal role in a healthy diet because they are an important source of energy, providing nourishment to every cell and organ in the body, especially the brain, which needs a constant stream of carb fuel to perform optimally. That said, not all carbohydrates are created equal, meaning that quality of carbs trumps quantity when it comes to good health *and* weight control.

Simple carbs, the kind found in highly processed and refined foods (sugar, flours, and other whites), are digested quickly, which causes a rapid surge of blood sugar. For this reason, they are considered high-glycemic foods. The addictive foods you read about on page 98 fall into this category. They fight weight-loss efforts by forcing the pancreas to release insulin in order to bring blood sugar back down. When this happens, excess sugar is stored as fat.

Healthier complex carbs, the type found in whole foods (those described in Principle No. 1) do the opposite. When you eat complex carbs, blood sugar rises gradually and insulin is released slowly, slowing down digestion and prolonging satiety. Which brings me to Brain-Powered Pointer No. 15:

**The body performs best when blood sugar is
kept relatively constant.**

The way to keep blood sugar in check is by choosing foods that have the least impact on blood sugar and insulin. The easiest and most accurate way to stay away from carbohydrates that do your weight-control efforts the most harm is to eat ones with a low to moderate glycemic load.

Foods with a low glycemic load (0-10):

- Beans and legumes, including chickpeas, kidney beans, black beans, lentils, and pinto beans

- Bran-based cereals (but watch for added sugars)

- Fruits

- Vegetables

Foods with a medium glycemic load (11–20):

- Barley (pearled)
- Brown rice
- Bulgur
- Fruit juices without added sugar
- Oatmeal
- Rice cakes
- Wheat berries
- Whole grain breads
- Whole grain pasta

In case you're curious: Glycemic load is a mathematical formula in which you multiply a particular food's glycemic index (a numerical value of how rapidly blood sugar rises on a scale of 0–100) by the number of net carbs (total carbs minus dietary fiber) in one serving. You can easily search the Internet for low to moderate glycemic load foods and come up with a long list of great options.

Principle No. 6: Be Mindful of Your Fat Consumption Every Day

Fat is not the scourge that doctors and nutritionists once thought it to be. This is due to the overwhelming mountain of evidence showing that certain types of fats—specifically monounsaturated fats, such as olive, canola, and nut oils, and polyunsaturated fats, such as safflower and sunflower oils—promote health by protecting us against life-threatening diseases, such as heart disease and certain forms of cancer. Too much saturated fat, the kind found in butter and marbled meat, is still linked to increased risk of certain health problems.

What hasn't changed about fat, however, is the fact that its calories can add up much too quickly. A gram of fat contains more than twice as many calories (9) as protein and carbohydrates (which each contain 4). This is the primary reason why you should never go overboard on fat no matter how good a certain fat may be for you. It just doesn't make good weight-loss *or* weight-maintenance sense. Just 1 tablespoon of any type of cooking oil is around 120 calories and 12 grams of fat, and you haven't eaten anything solid yet!

Fat serves a purpose in weight loss and weight maintenance because it helps you feel full quicker. That is a good thing. However, you have to be mindful of your intake because fat calories add up fast. One of the biggest problems I see is that people who "diet" tend to restrict one thing and compensate by overeating another. For example, people on low-carbohydrate diets tend to compensate for the lack of fruits, grains, and starches by eating more fat in the form of cheeses, sauces, and dressings. Overconsumption of *any* food or food group is not sound nutrition.

We love fat because it helps to liven up our food. We cook in it and spread it on sandwiches; we pour high-fat dressings over salads and sauces over meats and poultry. When it comes to fat, it is so easy to overdo it, which is why you must be mindful about how much you are actually eating. Make sure you know what a portion of fat really looks like. Are you sautéing your vegetables in a pool of olive oil, cooking your chicken in butter, and then putting some more fat on your pasta? You might be doing really well with your food choices, but overdoing fat without ever really meaning to. Fat is not the enemy—overconsumption of it is.

To keep a lid on your fat intake, always use a measuring spoon when sautéing and making dressings and sauces. Reduce your reliance on cooking oils by using cooking sprays and nonstick pans for browning. Always ask for your dressings and sauces on the side so you can control the amount you consume, especially in a restaurant. I have seen many salads featured on restaurant menus that contain as many calories and fat as a porterhouse steak. For example, a chicken Caesar salad may sound like a great idea but most varieties served in restaurants can run 600 to 800 calories or even more. This is why you need to be your own food advocate when dining out. Don't be afraid to ask questions!

When your diet is focused on nutritious whole foods and the other principles in this plan, and you are mindful about limiting added fat to your food, it is impossible to eat too much fat. Your total fat intake should be naturally low enough, leaving you plenty of room to fill up on flavorful foods you can actually chew.

There is only one type of fat you should avoid with diligence: trans fats. This man-made fat is just as bad for you as any other artificial food source and may still be lurking in some packaged foods. There has been such an uproar on the danger of trans fats and their contribution to obesity and the risk of life-threatening diseases, they have been all but eliminated from most products made in this country.

In addition to the healthy oils already mentioned, you can find quality fat in the following foods:

- Avocados and avocado oil
- Fatty fish, such as salmon and tuna
- Flaxseeds
- Nuts, including almonds, hazelnuts, peanuts, pecans, and walnuts by a small handful

Principle No. 7: Maximize Your Daily Fiber Intake

Eating plenty of dietary fiber is both a good health practice and an excellent weight-control strategy. Studies show that people who eat the most fiber tend to have a healthier body weight. One study found that people who ate no differently, except for increasing their fiber intake, lost as much weight as people who went on a rigid low-fat diet.

There is nothing magical about fiber that promotes weight loss. It doesn't help you burn fat or increase your metabolism. Rather, it helps your weight-loss and weight-control efforts because of what it doesn't do well. Fiber is not easily digestible, so it slows the release and absorption of glucose, making you feel fuller longer.

Fiber comes in two varieties. Insoluble fiber, the type found in wheat and many fruits and vegetables, primarily helps remove waste from your body. Soluble fiber, the type found in oats and beans, collects water as it goes through your system and takes unwanted substances such as cholesterol out of the body with it. All foods contain both kinds but are richer in one.

It doesn't really matter what type of fiber you eat as long as you get more of it in your diet. Sadly, for many people, this is a tall order. Most Americans eat less than half the 25 to 30 grams they should be getting on a daily basis to promote good health and weight control. However, you'll fix that quite handily when you focus on eating nutrient-dense whole foods. It's part of the synergy of the 10 Principles of Healthy Eating. Some of the best and tastiest sources of fiber include:

- Beans
- Berries
- Legumes
- Lentils
- Nuts

- Oats and oatmeal
- Pasta (whole grain)
- Popcorn (air-popped)
- Seeds
- Whole grain breads and crackers

Principle No. 8: Practice Portion Control

Food marketers are masters of delusion, and they have deluded the public about what a serving size is supposed to be. The reason most people get into caloric trouble is because they have an exaggerated view of portion size. This is reality: A 20-ounce bottle of cola is really 2½ servings, a 24-ounce porterhouse found on a steakhouse menu should serve a family of six, and a typical plate of pasta sold in an Italian restaurant is big enough for four people. That's a lot of over-the-top calories!

Lots of items cast before our eyes as normal are not even close, like double cheeseburgers, deep-deep-dish pizzas, triple-dip ice cream cones, salads oozing with blue cheese dressing, and oversized dessert specials.

One lesson that comes with self-monitoring is getting a grasp on serving size, and it's an important one. When you use a calorie-tracking app, it almost always gives you a caloric measure by serving size—usually ½ cup for most vegetables, fruits, and pastas, and 3 ounces for meat, fish, or other protein.

In Principle No. 3, I alluded to the possibility that you may not always have to be beholden to counting calories. The foods we favor we tend to eat over and over, so as you move forward you should get to the point where you know your calories almost by heart and serving size by sight. However, until you get there and know you can do it with confidence, get yourself a food scale and measuring cups and spoons and put them to use. Here's the rule of thumb on serving sizes:

Food	Amount	Visual
Beverages	8 ounces	Clenched fist
Cereals (cold)	1 cup	2 cupped handfuls
Salads	1 cup	2 cupped handfuls

Food	Amount	Visual
Soups	1 cup	2 cupped handfuls
Stews	1 cup	2 cupped handfuls
Beans	½ cup	1 handful
Cereals (hot)	½ cup	1 handful
Cottage cheese	½ cup	1 handful
Fruit salad	½ cup	1 handful
Grains	½ cup	1 handful
Yogurt	½ cup	1 handful
All meats, poultry, game, and fish	3 ounces	Palm of the hand
Dressings and condiments	2 tablespoons	2 thumbs
Butters and oils	1 tablespoon	1 thumb

Principle No. 9: Never Say "Never" to the Foods You Crave

Just say "almost never." People who have Healthy Obsession don't live in absolutes. That's because it's impossible and it doesn't leave any room for fun or adventure. It's unthinkable that you should live the rest of your life without indulging once in a while in an "off-plan" food. That includes even now when you're trying to lose weight and adopt a lifestyle of healthy eating.

That's right. You should never think of *any* food as being off-limits. Thinking this way can psychologically lead to rebellion. For instance, I can't honestly tell you the last time I had a doughnut. It's not because I've said to myself, "I'm never going to eat a doughnut again," it's because any time I've been faced with the choice of a doughnut or no doughnut, I've simply said, "I choose not to today." And over time, that's grown into not having eaten a doughnut in a very long time. It's not that I consider doughnuts, or anything for that matter, off-limits. I just feel that eating something else serves me much better. This is the way I'd like you to think. When faced with an off-plan food, consider the consequence of eating it. Which brings me to Brain-Powered Pointer No. 16:

The food is not the issue. The issue is
what the food does to your goals.

It's a simple fact. There are foods that will lead you toward weight loss and maintaining a healthy weight, and there are foods that will challenge your goals. It's all up to you. This is *your* program. I am not going to tell you what you can't eat, but you need to know that you will not succeed in weight loss if you regularly indulge in foods outside of the margins I've already defined as nutritious whole foods.

Here's the bottom line: You don't have to give up the foods you love. If you can't image life without ever eating a plate of chicken wings again, then have your chicken wings. Just eat less of them and only on a rare occasion. When the time comes that you find yourself tempted to go off plan, do so only if you can adhere to the following:

- You can partake while still staying on plan, meaning you are able to eat a reasonable amount and then move on. If, as the saying goes, you can't eat just one potato chip, then don't even try. Consider the food off-limits until you're comfortable knowing you can have a taste and move on.

- You can do so without reverting back to your old cognitive distortions. You must have the confidence to counter any thinking error that could sneak its way back into your mind—which means you won't say "I blew it" and find yourself in a weeklong binge.

- You plan for it ahead of time and limit the amount. Let your Wise Mind rule.

- You enlist your favorite Dealing Skills if you feel the urge for more.

- You don't indulge in something special as a reward for anything, especially for reaching a weight-loss milestone. This means not justifying your choice by saying "I deserve this." Instead, just acknowledge the truth—"I want this"—and consider the consequences.

- You never keep foods you're trying to avoid in the house. Having to make a special trip to indulge might give you pause while you ask yourself, "Is it really worth it?"

Here's the payoff for keeping these foods at arm's length almost all the time: You're going to desire them less and less. Studies in human behavior show that food preferences can change over time. The more you make healthy choices and the less you eat the foods you crave, the less you're going to want them.

Principle No. 10: Love Foods That Love You Back

This is not a journey of deprivation; consider it a journey of exploration. People tell me all the time that they are amazed at the large variety of food choices out there when they start eating according to these 10 principles. I trust you will have the same experience. Just always be mindful that your interest, willingness, and success at following this healthy foods plan will have a great deal to do with your mind-set, which brings me to Brain-Powered Pointer No. 17:

> Stay focused on the foods that serve you
> and not on the foods you want to avoid.

If you're like a lot of people, you've told yourself countless times that you're "going to start eating healthier." We all *want* that, right? Only it didn't happen—not really, anyway. The reason it didn't happen is because the pledge "to eat healthier" is just too vague. It's what is called a "soft goal," something you'll learn more about when you get to Step 8. To make the goal a reality, you have to get more to the point: *How* are you going to eat in order to make your diet healthy, and *what* are you going to eat?

Go back to the lists of foods in Principles No. 1, 5, and 7 and review all the healthy choices. Many of them are just categories. Take beans, for example. There are dozens of varieties of beans. How many kinds of beans do you eat? Navy, pinto, or kidney maybe? Expand your healthy options by exploring other types of beans, such as black, adzuki, fava, chickpeas, or, my favorite, lentils. Same with berries, nuts, and fruits. The varieties go on and on. Go to a health food market and you'll find aisle upon aisle of greens and other colorful vegetables. The richer they are in color, the more nutritious they are. What looks interesting? What would you like to try? Healthy foods number in the hundreds, and each one offers you the opportunity to learn to love a food that's going to love you back.

Mental Resilience Technique: How to Just Say No

Here's a positive eating habit to practice before each meal and snack and every time you get the urge to eat the wrong food or overindulge. Ask yourself these two questions:

1. Will I feel guilty, frustrated, or disappointed after eating this?

2. If the answer is yes, ask yourself this, as it is important: Am I okay with eating it anyway?

You'd be surprised how many people tell me that this simple mental exercise keeps them on the straight and narrow. They decide "No, I am NOT okay with that!" and just move on.

Now it's time to start thinking about composing your new healthy foods plan. It starts with examining and then doing a quick critique of your current food customs. Same goes with your typical methods of preparation. Let's say you love chicken and eat it several times a week. Great choice. Give it a check. But what cuts do you favor? Skinless breasts and thighs are both good choices. Fried wings probably won't get you to your goals— X it out. How do you prepare your chicken? If you take breast tenders and coat them in bread crumbs and fry them in oil, you're adding too many calories that offer you little in terms of nutrition—X it out. Decide instead to experiment with other methods, such as grilling and poaching. You get the idea.

Like most people, I like eggs because they are so good for you. I love hard-cooked eggs and always have them on hand for a quick snack or to add some protein to a lunchtime salad. How about you? If your relationship with eggs is all about omelets, examine them for quality. Switching, for example, from a western omelet to a vegetable omelet shouldn't be difficult.

Most people have a core diet limited to 20 to 30 base foods, including snacks. Think about your current diet and identify the 20 foods you eat most frequently. Write them down in the space below, in your journal, or download

"My Whole Foods Diet Plan" from my Web site, www.elizakingsford.com. If the food fits in any of the healthy food categories described previously, give it a check. If not, mark it with an X.

My Top 20 Foods		Method of Preparation		Healthier Prep Option
1.				
2.				
3.				
4.				
5.				
6.				
7.				
8.				
9.				
10.				
11.				
12.				
13.				
14.				
15.				
16.				
17.				
18.				
19.				
20.				

Next, go back to the lists in Principles No. 1, 5, and 7 and identify 20 healthy foods you'd like to explore as you embark on your new healthy food plan. Organize it just like the nutrient-dense food plate I described in Principle No. 1—half vegetables and fruits, leaning more toward the veggies; one-quarter grains, and one-quarter protein. Be open-minded. Even if you think you don't like, say, quinoa or Brussels sprouts, be willing to try them again. Maybe what you didn't like about them was the way they were prepared or what you were eating them with.

Before filling this in, give it a lot of thought. Visit a health foods store or a health-conscious supermarket. Talk to friends and acquaintances who you know enjoy healthy eating and cooking. What might they recommend you try? Better yet, find a partner or two who is interested in embarking on this journey with you. Turn it into a New Healthy Foods Club where you get together each week to discuss your new discoveries in healthy eating and exchange ideas and recipes.

Consider this list a work in progress, one that is always changing and expanding.

Vegetables

1. _____
2. _____
3. _____
4. _____
5. _____
6. _____

Fruits

1. _____
2. _____
3. _____
4. _____

Grains

1. _____
2. _____
3. _____
4. _____
5. _____

Protein

1. _____
2. _____
3. _____
4. _____
5. _____

This is your opportunity to design your own plan—the only person dictating what you should eat is *you*. Nobody can stick to a diet in which some expert dictates what you must and must not eat, at least not over the long haul. The same can be said about exercise. You don't need me to tell you that you should exercise or what type of exercise you should do. To find out what will help you get more movement into your life, see Step 7.

HOW THESE PRINCIPLES TRANSLATE TO REALITY

You might still be wondering what a typical day eating according to these principles looks like. Here is a three-day example. These menus, which contain minimal to no processed foods, come in at around 1,500 to 1,800 calories, at least 30 grams of fiber, and 30 to 50 grams of fat, most of which are healthy fats.

Day 1

BREAKFAST

Two-egg omelet with red potatoes, feta cheese, diced tomatoes, and garlic

½ cup natural plain yogurt with blueberries

Herbal tea or coffee with milk and honey, if needed

SNACK

Apple with natural almond butter (no added or artificial ingredients)

LUNCH

Homemade vegetable soup

Pita pocket sandwich with sliced tomatoes, avocado, turkey, hummus, and whole grain pita bread

Field greens with no more than a tablespoon of olive oil and some lemon

Unsweetened iced tea

DINNER

Jumbo shrimp baked with a drizzle of olive oil, seasoning of your choice, and served with lemon wedges

½ cup brown rice pilaf with peas, pancetta, and onions

Roasted asparagus sprinkled with Parmesan cheese

Sliced tomatoes

Poached pear

SNACK

Pretzels, low-fat popcorn, or whole fruit

Day 2

BREAKFAST

1 cup old-fashioned natural oatmeal with sliced banana, berries, and slivered almonds made with almond milk

1 slice whole grain toast with cottage cheese

Coffee or tea

SNACK

Fresh peach and ¼ cup cashews

LUNCH

Homemade chicken salad with diced chicken, avocado, apple, celery, onion, herbs, salt, and pepper

Mixed greens with olive oil, Himalayan pink sea salt, and lemon

DINNER

3 ounces grilled flank steak

Spinach salad with sliced hard-cooked egg, mushrooms, sliced red onions, sliced strawberries, and walnuts with balsamic vinaigrette

Steamed green beans with toasted garlic and almonds

Glass red wine, if desired

SNACK

Apple slices with 2 teaspoons all-natural peanut butter

Day 3

BREAKFAST

High-fiber, no-sugar-added whole grain cereal, such as Bob's Red Mill Muesli, with milk

Cantaloupe

SNACK

Two hard-cooked eggs

LUNCH

Two chicken tacos with sautéed bell peppers and onions and dollops of tomato salsa, sour cream, and guacamole on corn tortillas

Mixed greens and orange slices with balsamic vinegar

DINNER

Poached salmon with lemon butter sauce

Quinoa with dried cherries and chopped walnuts

Steamed broccoli and cauliflower

SNACK

Handful of mixed nuts

I do not like to tell people what to eat—that's just putting them on a diet. Besides, if I did, you probably wouldn't like some of the things I tell you to eat, so you'd just stop doing what I suggest altogether. Rather, what's more important—and actually, very important—is *learning* how to create a healthy menu for yourself, equipped with all the foods you enjoy and are willing to eat.

META MENTORING WITH ELIZA

"Designing My Own Weight-Loss Plan Was Empowering!"

Some of my clients are surprised and a bit uneasy (at first) when I tell them to design their own weight-loss plan based on the 10 Principles of Healthy Eating. The conversation with them typically goes along the same lines as the talk I had with my client, Barry, who was one of the most reluctant of them all. Similar thoughts may be going through your mind. My hope is that you'll discover, as Barry did, that "designing my own weight-loss plan was empowering."

Barry: Okay, so I should eat what I want as long as I stick with nutrient-dense whole foods and keep calories to what works for me. I get it, but that's just too vague for me. I'll screw it up. I'd rather you tell me what to eat three times a day. To me, that's what's easy, and it's the way I've always done it in the past.

Me: What you just said, "the way I've always done it in the past," how'd that go for you? I'm guessing not well or you wouldn't be here with me now. That didn't work for you in the past, and it's not the way you're eating now.

Barry: (chuckles) You're right, it didn't work. There was no way I could keep it up. Most of the diets I've been on, I really didn't like the food all that much. Some were better suited to me than others—loved the low carb. I stuck with them, but I couldn't wait until they were over.

Me: Barry, but that's the point. When the diet "ends," you go back to all your old eating habits. You need to design your own healthy eating plan around foods that you like *and* that are good for you, then change your thinking habits so these foods become your new eating habit. I could do a list of foods for you, but you probably wouldn't like the foods I'd pick, so what's the point? If you want to lose weight and keep it off, you need to adopt a healthy eating style based on the kinds of foods that you like and can continue to eat forever.

Barry: But I like cheeseburgers. (He teased with a thin smile.) I could eat *them* forever.

Me: Okay, so let's talk cheeseburgers then. Eating a typical restaurant-style cheeseburger, is that getting you closer or farther away from your goals?

Barry: Farther, obviously.

Me: Okay. That said, take the words "can't eat" out of your vocabulary. That means you *can* eat a cheeseburger. The choice is always yours. You just need to be mindful of the consequences: How is it going to affect your plan and your goals?

Barry: I know. The consequences are big. You can't lose weight eating cheeseburgers.

Me: Well, you can't lose weight eating cheeseburgers all the time, but if you love cheeseburgers, you don't have to tell yourself you can't ever eat one again. There are ways you can have your cheeseburger and still be on plan.

Barry: I know. Immediately get back on plan the next meal. See, I'm a good learner. (He smiles.)

Me: Yes, that. But there are also ways to reduce the harm in eating a cheeseburger. For example, you could pile it with fresh vegetables, instead of cheese and fried onions, and save yourself a lot of unneeded calories and fat. You could share it with someone or have it cut in half and then only eat half. You can cut your habit of eating burgers every week to once a month or once every other month. Plan when you're going to have a cheeseburger so you can plan your other meals for that day around it so you don't overeat. You could experiment and order a turkey burger or a veggie burger or a bean burger when you get a burger craving. I bet you'll be surprised that after being away from cheeseburgers for a while, you won't be craving them like you used to.

Barry: Okay. I'm getting it. But I'm still not comfortable with this designing-your-own stuff. I don't know anything about nutrition.

Me: If you stick to nutrient-dense whole foods and design your plate according to the guidelines in Principle 1, you don't have to be worried about nutrition. You'll be getting plenty of nutrition and fiber and other good-for-you nutrients.

Barry: How will I know?

Me: Tracking what you eat is crucial to staying on plan. You can't manage if you don't monitor. The app I told you to download will track all the nutritional data you need. You're doing that, aren't you?

Barry: Sort of, but it gives me bad news. I ate a tuna hoagie the other day and found it was 920 calories. Tuna's on my list of lovable foods!

Me: Sure, tuna is on your list. But is tuna mixed with mayonnaise, topped with cheese and more mayo on a huge white-bread hoagie roll? I doubt it. If you had looked it up *before* ordering, you would have saved yourself the frustration of realizing that this sandwich does not serve you. It's an important tool. You probably would have been better off with a cheeseburger!

Barry: I knew you'd come around to my way of thinking. Only kidding! I know. I should make my own tuna salad so I can control the fat and calories.

Me: Your job is to fill your plate with nutrient-dense whole foods like we've talked about, foods that are closest to their natural form as much of the time as possible. When you are choosing what to eat or what to make for dinner, you want to always ask yourself if you are choosing nutrient-dense whole foods or if your foods are processed. Does that sound doable?

Barry: Well, yeah, you make it sound simple enough.

Me: That's where you start—simple. Monitor your food intake and choose nutrient-dense whole foods. Once you get comfortable there, we can start to look at tweaking your food intake, looking at overall calories or certain macronutrients. But for now, let's start simple.

Barry: Okay that helps. Don't get too overwhelmed.

Me: Then go back to the 10 food principles and start to see where else you can incorporate some changes. Are you getting enough fiber? Are you choosing complex rather than simple carbohydrates? Are you being mindful of your fat intake? Remember, this is like a marathon, not a sprint. This is about adopting a new lifestyle, not a diet. So be patient and give yourself lots of space. Start simple.

Barry had a hard time at first getting started on the program, but only because he was filled with self-doubt about his ability to do it. He had been told by numerous diet books what to eat, what recipes to follow, what foods were off-limits, and what foods he could have. My goal was to teach Barry how to make his own food decisions and how to evaluate whether they were serving him. Armed with my food principles and his trusty self-monitoring device, Barry set off to find out what the best plan was for him. It worked remarkably well. He says that he feels more empowered now than he ever felt on any of his previous diets.

Make Room for More Movement in Your Life

A lot of fitness and weight-loss experts say that it's a challenge to motivate people to get out and exercise. That's not my experience. I find it *impossible* to motivate someone to exercise. The reason: Lasting motivation can only come from within. Sure, I can get someone to join in on a fitness class most days, as I can be pretty persuasive. But for sustained success, you have to be able to motivate yourself.

I'm not going to lecture you about the importance of exercise, because I am certain you already know how essential it is. I could spend the next several pages laying out the scientific evidence showing that exercise can help:

- Improve executive function, the area of the brain that regulates our ability to make decisions, plan, and exert the positive thinking power we need to overcome bad habits.

- Increase your ability to lose weight, because it stokes your calorie burn and keeps it up there for hours afterward.

- Counter the decline in basal metabolic rate caused by calorie restriction.

- Protect and build stronger bones and increase muscle mass.

- Decrease appetite, boost energy, perk up your mood, and improve sleep.

- Reduce your risks of heart disease, diabetes, certain kinds of cancers, dementia, and depression.

- Improve quality of life into old age and even help increase longevity.

Only I'm going to bypass that. No matter how convincing the research is, I doubt it will be enough to get you to a gym or on a walking path for more than a few weeks or months, if at all, if you aren't self-motivated. What I am going to

do is give you what I know works best for success over the long haul—the tools
to motivate yourself. Which brings me to Brain-Powered Pointer No. 18:

Movement does even more for mental well-being
than it does for physical health.

TIC-TOC Your Way into an Active Lifestyle

This activity is designed to get out of the mental rut that keeps us
from being more active. It's called the TIC-TOC Technique: TIC, meaning task-interfering cognitions, and TOC, which stands for task-
oriented cognitions. TICs that lead to TOCs can lead to task-oriented
actions.

TICs are the excuses we use that prevent us from doing something we have a desire to do but can't find the motivation to make
happen. TOCs are a response using nonjudgmental thinking. Here's
an example:

TIC: I'd like to join the hiking club in my community, but I'm too out of
shape and know I won't be able to keep up.

COGNITIVE DISTORTION(S): black-and white thinking; overgeneralization

TOC: It may be hard at first, but I'm not getting anywhere just sitting
here. I've worked my way through hard things before.

TASK-ORIENTED ACTION: Everybody has to start somewhere, and they
must have newcomers all the time. I am going to call and inquire about
joining a beginner's group.

Now, it's your turn. If you lead a sedentary lifestyle, meaning you
are like most Americans and only move an average of about 5,000
steps a day (a little over 2 miles), you have been wallowing in a lot of
excuses that are nothing more than TICs. Recognize them for what
they are and turn them into TOCs. In the following spaces, think of the
top five excuses you use for not being more physically active or that
prevent you from getting involved in organized physical activities. Or
you can download the worksheet called "TIC-TOC Technique" from
my Web site, www.elizakingsford.com, and put them in your journal.

When it comes to thinking about getting more physically active, cognitive distortions run rampant. "My life is crazy-busy" or "I'm too embarrassed to go to a gym—people will make fun of me behind my back" or "I'm so out of shape, it's useless" or "Are you kidding—me in shorts and a sports bra?" These are excuses you've told yourself so often, you've convinced yourself they are true.

1. **TIC:** _____

   Cognitive distortion: _____

   TOC: _____

   Task-oriented action: _____

2. **TIC:** _____

   Cognitive distortion: _____

   TOC: _____

   Task-oriented action: _____

3. **TIC:** _____

   Cognitive distortion: _____

   TOC: _____

   Task-oriented action: _____

4. **TIC:** _____

   Cognitive distortion: _____

   TOC: _____

   Task-oriented action: _____

5. **TIC:** _____

   Cognitive distortion: _____

   TOC: _____

   Task-oriented action: _____

Only now, hopefully, not so much. Now that you've worked your way through Steps 3, 4, and 5, you should be able to see this type of thinking as nothing more than cognitive distortions working overtime. You've been overgeneralizing, jumping to conclusions, and living in can't, shouldn't, and mustn't thinking. Change your automatic negative thoughts to positive counter thoughts and your motivation will be much easier to find. "Taking that brisk walk was exhilarating!" "That workout was awesome." That's what people with Healthy Obsession think because that's what exercise really feels like.

So, let's give you the opportunity to find out for yourself. As you start to experience the physical benefits of a more active lifestyle, you'll begin to see your life with more mental clarity and your mental distortions will be much easier to tame—"I didn't really lose much weight last week, but, hey, my belt's in a notch. Where's my gym bag?!" It's mental synergy at its best.

PLACING VALUE ON MOTIVATION

Losing weight or, say, running 10 miles isn't easy. It doesn't happen on its own. Having the desire to do it isn't enough to make it happen, which brings me to Brain-Powered Pointer No. 19:

> The only way to get physically active is to activate the behaviors that will make it happen.

It means you have to be persistent in overcoming the obstacles that will get in your way—"I'm so intimidated at my Pilates class, but if I get in the front of the class, I won't see how well everybody else is doing!"—and possess the mental stamina to keep going when the going gets tough—"I'm too tired and my muscles ache, but I know the exercise will invigorate me." It takes:

- **Activation:** Make the decision to pursue a new behavior. Example: "I am going to walk for 30 minutes every morning before my day begins."

- **Intensity:** This is the vigor that will be required to attain the goal. Example: "I will have to go to bed a half hour earlier and set my alarm 45 minutes earlier, which will give me the time to dress and undress for the walk."

- **Persistence:** This is the continued effort that will be required to over-come obstacles. For example, "I have an early appointment tomorrow, so I will take my walking wear with me to work and walk over my lunch hour."

Now, think about what you would like to do to get more physical activity in your life and what you must require of yourself to get there. Fill in the blanks below or download the document called "Activity Commitment" for your notebook or journal from my Web site, www.elizakingsford.com.

1. The type of activity I want to pursue (activation):

   _____

   _____

   What will be required of me to make it happen (intensity):

   _____

   _____

   What I must do to keep it ongoing (persistence):

   _____

   _____

2. The type of activity I want to pursue (activation):

   _____

   _____

   What will be required of me to make it happen (intensity):

   _____

   _____

   What I must do to keep it ongoing (persistence):

   _____

   _____

3. The type of activity I want to pursue (activation):

   _____

   _____

What will be required of me to make it happen (intensity):

_____

_____

What I must do to keep it ongoing (persistence):

_____

_____

This is an ideal start, but it won't necessarily get you to the finish line. You still need the motivation to make it happen. Motivation isn't something that is handed to you, nor is it something you can buy. It comes from within.

There are two types of motivation that drive your desire to achieve a goal—what we call extrinsic and intrinsic motivation. Extrinsic motivation comes from outside yourself. It's what you're going to get in return for doing something, the end goal that motivation will achieve. "I want to get back into my size 8 jeans." "I want to be able to wear a bikini this summer." "I want to have the flat abs I see on the cover of those men's magazines." It's the reward, the incentive.

Intrinsic motivation comes from inside yourself: "Exercise gives me energy and mental stamina. It makes me feel terrific." When you have intrinsic motivation, achieving the task is its own reward. It's engaging in a behavior (exercise) because it is personally rewarding. The way it makes you feel is more important than fitting back in your size 8 jeans. Which brings me to Brain-Powered Pointer No. 20:

> **Extrinsic motivation will get you started, but it takes intrinsic motivation to get you to the finish.**

It's why I said at the beginning of this step that motivation must come from within. Studies and anecdotal evidence show that extrinsic motivation alone can actually backfire. For example, studies found that children who were rewarded for doing something they already enjoyed, such as playing with a certain toy, eventually became less interested in pursuing the activity when an award was attached to it. In other words, you are more likely to stick with exercise if you are doing it because it makes you feel terrific (intrinsic) than if you are doing it so you look terrific in a bikini (extrinsic). If your motivation to exercise comes *only* from wanting to lose 30 pounds or to look terrific in a bikini, then making slow progress toward reaching your goal can easily lead to decreased interest in exercise.

People who lapse at exercise frequently lack intrinsic motivation. This doesn't mean you can't or shouldn't have extrinsic motivation. For many people, it's a great way to get started, but you also need intrinsic motivation to make it stick.

FINDING YOUR INTRINSIC MOTIVATOR

I bet exercise is not new to you. You've probably tried it in the past and dropped out for some reason. You may even have given it a try several times. The reason you didn't follow through is because intrinsic motivation just wasn't there. Here is how you can take the emphasis off your extrinsic motivation and pursue an intrinsic one:

- Focus on the journey (your incremental accomplishments) more than the outcome (fitting into those jeans): "How much farther did I go today? How did it make me feel?"

- Praise the effort (your hard work) rather than the progress (the jeans almost fit): "Wow, I'm now running 3 miles, and today I started resistance training."

- Assess your efforts so you can fine-tune your motivation. "Running five times a week is making my knees hurt. I'm going to run three times a week every other day and walk the days in between, with one day of rest."

What would intrinsic motivation look like for you? For example, you might say:

1. I want to run in a 5K race, which I never thought I could do.

2. I want to be able to do two flights of stairs without getting out of breath.

3. I want to be able to easily get down on the floor to play with my grandkids.

In the space below or in your notebook or journal, list five intrinsic reasons for you to exercise, even if you're not feeling them right now. Or go to the document called "Intrinsic Motivators" on my Web site, www.elizakingsford.com.

My Intrinsic Reasons to Put More Movement in My Life

1. _____

2. _____

3. _____

4. _____

5. _____

GEARING UP FOR MORE MOVEMENT

When I talk about movement, I am not just talking about participating in an aerobic activity or working with weights. If you're like a lot of people, you'll welcome this is as good news. Even if you don't go to a gym (or aren't ready yet), it is important to purposefully and mindfully get your body more active starting right now. Which brings me to Brain-Powered Pointer No. 21:

The only fitness activity you will stick with is one that you will enjoy.

My definition of physical activity is any movement that enables your body to burn more calories than it does at rest. This includes parking at the back of the lot so you have to walk farther, delivering a message to a colleague in person instead of sending an e-mail, skipping the drive-thru and actually ordering your morning coffee on foot, shopping the aisles of the supermarket instead of calling in your order, gardening and mowing your own grass, cleaning the house yourself, walking the kids to the bus stop instead of driving them, riding your bicycle on errands instead of taking the car, and walking, walking, walking every opportunity you get. Make the commitment and mindfully look for ways you can work in more steps every day.

Walking is a great activity, especially if you aren't able to jog or power walk. It's something most all of us can do. In fact, it is the only type of exercise I am

Get Off Your But

We all try to talk ourselves out of doing something that's going to take a little (or more) effort to meet our goals. It's never more true than when it comes to building more activity into your life. Next time it happens to you, enlist the But-Rebuttal Method, an exercise designed to help you trace the thinking patterns you use to talk yourself out of doing what you really want to do or know you should be doing.

Here's an example of how it works. Trace your own internal arguments in the space below, in your journal, or download the document called "But-Rebuttal Method" from my Web site.

But	But Rebuttal
I really should go to the gym, but I'm just not in the mood.	But I'll feel more like it once I get started.
But I'm too tired to go to the gym, and my muscles still hurt from last time.	But I could at least get up and take a brisk long walk.
But I'm watching golf, and it's a good match.	But that's not going to burn any calories, and the match will be on for hours. I won't miss much.
But I'm feeling too lazy, and walking is getting so boring.	But that can't be true. I haven't missed my goal to go 10,000 steps a day in 2 weeks.

My Buts and Rebuttals

But	But Rebuttal
1.	1.
2.	2.
3.	3.
4.	4.
5.	5.
1.	1.
2.	2.
3.	3.
4.	4.
5.	5.

going to ask you to pledge to start right away. I strongly recommend that you buy yourself a fitness tracker and commit to walking a minimum of 10,000 steps a day.

The 10,000 step program was initiated in 1996 as a federal endeavor to help get Americans more active by moving more. I love the whole idea because of the sneaky-cool way it builds in real exercise. Ten thousand steps is roughly 5 miles. Unless you are a waitperson, nurse, or fitness instructor, most people can't work in that kind of mileage in a typical day without making a concerted effort to tie on a pair of sneakers and go out for a walk.

Committing to 10,000 steps a day is a great way to incentivize yourself to get up out of your chair and take a walk around the block when you're bound to a desk all day. Or, better yet, get yourself out for a brisk 30-minute walk as a regular exercise routine. If you can't do 30 minutes in one shot, then try for 10 minutes three times a day. Studies show that three 10-minute bursts of energy offer the same health and fitness benefits as one 30-minute session.

In order to make it real exercise, walk as if you're late for an appointment. Bend your arms, keep them close to your body, make lose fists, and pump slightly. Getting your heart rate up is the way to improve cardiovascular fitness, which is important for all of us. And it will increase your calorie burn. Do it consistently, and it will help change your weight, your body, and your health.

Affirm to Walk 10,000 Steps

You will increase your chances of meeting your daily goal of 10,000 steps by writing an affirmation, such as:

I am capable of achieving what I set my mind to.

I am strong and continue to get stronger each day.

Now, come up with your own fitness affirmation (or use this one) and write it here or in your journal or notebook.

_____

_____

_____

_____

Recite it every morning when you awaken and repeat it every time you check in with your tracking device.

THE JOY OF ACTIVE LIVING

Exercise and physical activity are two different things. Exercise is a muscle-exerting effort that is planned, structured, purposeful, repetitive, and, most importantly, something you will strive to do at least three to five times per week. Examples include running, swimming, strength training, yoga, tennis, strenuous hiking, and most types of organized sports. Physical activity is any movement that enables your body to burn more calories than it would at rest. Examples include house cleaning, walking, gardening, and even taking the stairs to the seventh floor instead of the elevator.

Experience tells us that the only exercise that will work is something that fits into your lifestyle and your personal circumstances. For example, if you're a single parent with a full-time job and you live 20 miles from the closest gym, going to a Pilates class three times a week probably isn't going to last very long. However, working out with a Pilates class on your computer in the morning before the rest of the family gets up is more realistic.

Love baseball or basketball? Don't just watch it—play it. Most communities and local gyms have adult leagues set up for the purpose of offering both fun and exercise. If there isn't one in your community, get proactive and start one. Bowling and golfing may only offer brief spurts of energy, but at least they get you on your feet and doing something that's also social and enjoyable.

Experiment with different exercises, sports, classes, gyms, and recreational activities. Do so within the context of understanding your own limitations, tolerance, and functional capacity for exercise. Pick an activity in line with the Centers for Disease Control and Prevention's guidelines for physical fitness, weight loss, and weight control.

- Spend a minimum of 2½ hours a week doing moderate aerobic exercise, such as jogging, or 75 minutes of high-intensity exercise, such as running. Breaking up the exercise into shorter sessions is fine—this is a great way for overweight and obese individuals to begin. Some forms of exercise that may interest you include:

  - Basketball
  - Bicycling
  - Dancing
  - Golfing (without a cart)
  - Hiking
  - Jogging
  - Kayaking

- ○ Kickboxing
- ○ Pilates
- ○ Running
- ○ SCUBA diving
- ○ Skating
- ○ Skiing
- ○ Soccer
- ○ Step climbing
- ○ Swimming
- ○ Yoga
- ○ Zumba

- Engage in structured strength training that uses all the major muscle groups—legs, hips, back, abs, chest, shoulders, arms—at least twice a week. Strength training also includes weight lifting, the use of resistance bands, and doing pushups, pullups, and situps, in which your body weight furnishes the resistance. If you don't want to go public at a gym, you can do a workout in the privacy of your own home by signing up for any number of exercise videos available on the Internet. Two of my favorite sites are beachbody.com and dailyburn.com.

THE MOTIVATION BOOSTER

One of the best ways to help boost your motivation is by using a fitness tracker. I love these devices.

Fitness trackers have come a long way since the analog step-counting pedometers of 10 and even 5 years ago. Modern trackers use accelerometers, devices used to guide spaceflight, that monitor how far and how intensely you move daily. They also keep track of the calories you burn. Your steps, miles,

---

Mental Resilience Technique:
Issue a Challenge

Train your brain to recognize that there is more than one way to get moving. Issue a "step challenge" to your family or co-workers. It's simple: Whoever covers the most distance in the course of a week wins. I've found most people will step right up to the challenge because it sounds easy and fun. You can even offer a reward of your choice to the winner. For example, everyone throws $1 in a pot and the winner takes all. Or the winner is treated to a pair of movie tickets. Keep the reward small and fun, so it can be ongoing. Just make sure it doesn't involve food.

Stretch and Move

Here's a little feel-good exercise you can use anytime anywhere: Stand up and stretch. Arch your back and stretch your arms and fingers out wide. Hold that posture for a while and then let go. Now move your body all around to get the blood pumping. Clap your hands. Jump up and down. Now get a move on.

and calories show up on the screen of the device that you can either wear as a clip-on to your waistband or on your wrist as a watch. Some, like the Fitbit that I wear, can communicate with your smartphone, computer, or tablet and will keep track of the steps and miles you cover over time. Some are so sophisticated they can give you a readout on your weight, heart rate, blood oxygen, skin temperature, and perspiration. Wear it to bed and it will even monitor sleep time and quality. You can pay anywhere from $30 for the most basic device to more than $300 for the most sophisticated ones.

What I like best about fitness trackers is the encouragement they offer. Everyone I counsel and everybody who attends Wellspring Camps uses one, and most everybody loves it. They enjoy the immediate feedback it provides and the history it stores. It's like your own personal electronic diary.

Many trackers can even go one better by allowing you to social network with other people on the same path as you and get real-time feedback. This is a powerful benefit. Research shows that social support can be one of the biggest drivers of weight-loss and weight-control success. When people feel connected to others who share similar goals, it reinforces them to work harder to attain their goals.

There is one caveat you need to keep in mind when it comes to fitness trackers. The readout numbers they generate are only estimates based on the information you provided. You shouldn't take it as gospel, which brings me to Brain-Powered Pointer No. 22:

Exercise should never be used as an excuse to eat more.

I simply do not believe in it! Using a fitness device as a tracker to eat more can be a slippery slope. You need to know what is a normal amount of food for you on a daily basis and stick to it. It doesn't matter if you walked 7 miles touring

Paris or New York on your vacation. Stick to your routine and the eating habits you are trying to establish. Also, the calorie burn that a fitness app reports is moderately accurate at best. As I've already explained in Step 6, there are many factors that contribute to an individual's calorie burn, and it is impossible for any fitness tracker to account for them all.

The most useful way to look at your calorie burn is to compare it over time. As you get more comfortable with your fitness level, you should be able to increase the duration and intensity of your workouts. This is a much better way of letting you know that your calorie burn is increasing.

MAKE THE PLEDGE

Now it's time to make a pledge to give all this a try. Putting more movement and activity in your life is self-rewarding. The more active you become, the better you're going to feel, which brings me to Brain-Powered Pointer No. 23:

> Exercise alone does not lead to greater
> weight loss than dieting alone, but the two together
> is how you will achieve optimal success.

An active lifestyle and healthy eating go hand in hand to form a healthy lifestyle. You can't have one without the other. Doing one without the other will only slow your progress and possibly weaken your resolve. Studies show

---

Support System in Cyberspace

Research tells us that working out with someone else creates a social contract and motivates you to push harder and go longer. It also armors your commitment, because you not only are accountable to yourself, but you also can't let the other person down.

If you don't have a neighbor or friend to enlist in your exercise efforts, you can still take advantage of a different style of the buddy system in the virtual world. Find a workout video or exercise class on cable television and exercise along with it. Research at Michigan State University found that women who rode a stationary bicycle with a virtual partner worked harder, especially when the other person was more fit.

that formally committing to do something by putting it in writing increases your resolve to honor it. Make your pledge here, or download the document "Movement Pledge and Worksheet" from my Web site, www.elizakingsford .com, and keep it in your notebook or journal.

MY PLEDGE TO MOVE MORE

Starting _____ (fill in the date), I pledge to make every effort to walk 10,000 steps (about 5 miles) a day. By _____ (fill in a date), I will take up _____ as a repeated form of aerobic exercise.

    Then check in with yourself on a daily basis. This will create adherence and accountability. Each day can look something like this:

Day 1 (date): _____

What I did:

_____

_____

_____

_____

Length of time:

_____

_____

How I felt before I started:

_____

_____

_____

_____

How I felt when I was finished:

_____

_____

_____

_____

AIM FOR YOUR BEST

I am a self-described fitness maven. Exercise and activity are part of who I am. And I love it. I've been an athlete all my life. I get aerobic activity by hiking, biking, or running three to five times a week; working out at the gym three times a week; and teaching a cycling class once a week. I measure the shape I'm in not by the scale, but by my ability to run up the mountain that is practically in my backyard in Boulder, Colorado—it's my intrinsic motivating factor.

As much as I'm committed to keeping my schedule day by day and week by week, I know it is not always possible. Some days life gets too full, and I have to let go of a planned workout or run. The same will happen to you. When it does, plan for it with some type of compensation. For example, I travel a lot on business. On days I have to take long flights, I know I won't get in any formal exercise because of my packed schedule. But I will go out of my way to get in lots of extra steps by parking as far away as possible in the airport lot, walking the corridors of the terminal instead of sitting and reading or looking at my phone while waiting to board, and making sure I'm eating very healthy throughout the day.

Affirm to Do Your Best

Every day at about noon, ask yourself aloud, "Am I doing my best today?" Don't settle for "your best" being another day of sitting at your computer and then sitting on the couch at night. Be honest with yourself—"What is my best so far today?" If, by noon, your day isn't looking so good from a fitness angle, you still have time to turn it around; if it is, give yourself a pat on the back and keep on moving.

This is all to say that the only commitment you can make on a daily basis is to do the best you can do. Most likely you won't be able to work in 10,000 steps every single day, but when you do the best you can do, you won't let yourself down. Doing the best you can do is all about being prepared for the day ahead through planning and setting goals for yourself, which is where I am taking you next.

META MENTORING WITH ELIZA

She Couldn't Imagine Ever
Stepping Back into a Gym

Sally S. was a self-described "exercise nut" who ran over her lunch hour every day and took a step class after work 4 days a week. She said it kept her body trim, her complexion rosy, and her spirits high. Only that was 10 years ago. Now, at age 55, she sat in front of me 20 pounds overweight, glum, and, as she described, "full of flab." I was trying to help her find her way back to the gym and back to an active lifestyle.

Sally: It's not that I don't know I should exercise. I used to love to exercise, but I got away from it when I started my own business. It got beyond me. I did nothing but work, work, work to keep up. It had me so stressed. I was eating poorly and exercising intermittently. It got to the point where I stopped trying to do any kind of exercise 5 years ago. Now look at me. I tried running a few times, but with the hills where I live it's just too hard. I can't even make a half mile. So, I joined a health club with an indoor track 4 months ago, only I haven't even gone once.

Me: What's preventing you from going? I know that gym, and you paid a lot of money to join.

Sally: I know! I tell myself that all the time. I don't know why I can't make myself go. I just can't get motivated.

Me: You joined the club, so something motivated you to do that. What made you want to join?

Sally: I want to get back to looking and feeling like I used to.

Me: That's great. It says you're motivated. Looking like you used to is called extrinsic motivation. That's what gets you started. And wanting to feel great like you did when you used to exercise is called intrinsic motivation. It's what you need to get to where you want to be. So, what seems to be the problem?

Sally: Don't know. I packed my gym bag and drove to the gym three times already, but I couldn't get myself to go in.

Me: Okay, let's take an imaginary journey together. Let's say I'm in your car going to the gym with you. We get out, check in, go to the locker room, start to change. Okay so far?

Sally: Not really. I'm feeling self-conscious already and I'm not even really there. It's me, fat, with my big running shorts and oversized T-shirt. Everyone else is wearing shorts and sports bras. They look great.

Me: So? They look great. Fact. What about that is difficult for you?

Sally: I'm just too intimidated. I guess that's it. Everyone is fit and I'm not.

Me: How do you know they are all fit? Where does that fact come from? How do you know some of them aren't there for the first time, just like you? How do you know they don't feel just as intimidated by all of the shorts and sports bras? You're overgeneralizing. Now imagine we go to the track. What are you feeling?

Sally: Inhibited. All of these fit people zooming by me and me just plodding along, going too slow. Annoying them. Them wondering, "What does she think she's doing?" (she says with a sneer).

Me: They said that? Out loud?

Sally: No, no one *says* it. (She smiles a bit and rolls her eyes.)

Me: So how do you know they are thinking that? You can read their minds? How do you know they don't see you as just someone new, like they were once? You know, every single person on that track had their first time on the same track. Every single one of them had to start at the beginning at one time just like you. Here's the thing about other people. They are much more worried about themselves and their own workout to be caring about yours. They're paying attention to their own lives.

Sally: Guess you're right about that, but it doesn't make me feel any less intimidated now. They're running for a half hour or more. I probably won't make 5 minutes.

Me: You can make the distance. Why don't you try this: Run for 2 minutes, then walk for a minute. I bet you can do that for a half hour. You used to run all the time. Fitness tends to come back faster after a relapse. If you don't like what you're wearing, find something you'll feel good about wearing.

Sally took my advice and 3 months later reported that joining the gym was the best thing she had done for herself in a decade. "I forgot how runners are so encouraging to other runners, and they really gave me a lot of motivation," she said. "And you were right about the fitness coming back faster. I'm running for a full half hour every time I'm there and am aiming for an hour." And the scale? She rarely steps on it because she likes the way she looks and feels.

Set SMART Goals and Plans

Thinking smarter, eating better, moving more. How do you get it all to work in sync? By setting goals—not the long-term goal to lose x-amount of pounds in x-amount of time, but well-planned short-term goals that can be measured every day.

More than 50 studies show that setting specific "hard goals"—"I will choose nutrient-dense whole foods at each meal"—leads to better performance than do-your-best "soft" goals—"I want to lose some weight"—or no goals at all—"I sure wish I could lose some weight." Hard goals improve both effort and performance. Dieters, however, tend to make decisions in very haphazard ways—"I'm going on a vegetarian diet until I lose 30 pounds"—and that usually results in increased vulnerability to setbacks before the goal is achieved. It simply is not enough to vow I *will* lose 30 pounds by bathing suit season, no matter how determined you may be. There's also the reality: How are you going to get there?

To truly succeed, you need to direct your attention to the small-detail goals and not the big-picture goal. Losing weight is a journey, and like any journey you need a map and a plan to reach your destination. You wouldn't take off on a cross-country auto trip without a map and a plan, would you? Consider your daily goals like your innate GPS: Stick with it and you will get to your destination. Which brings me to Brain-Powered Pointer No. 24:

> If you don't aim for a target,
> you will never hit anything.

Setting specific daily goals enables you to live with intention, because every morning you wake up, you know exactly what you need to do that day.

For example:

1. I will walk 3 miles before work 3 times this week.

2. Tonight I'm going out for dinner with a friend and will only go someplace where I can eat fish.

3. Before each meal, I will practice this affirmation: I will eat only until I no longer feel hungry, so I stop before I'm too full.

When you don't consciously consider your hard goals, your mind tends to stray back to mental chatter, the negative pull that leads to thinking errors, which raises the risk of a setback. Like your GPS, your daily goals are always there to remind you to recalculate and get back on track. They become part of your new running tape that continually plays in your head, and they keep you focused on the win. Setting them should be as perfunctory as brushing your teeth.

THE POWER OF GOALS

The way to make a goal meaningful is to make sure it fits the acronym SMART, which stands for specific, measurable, attainable, realistic, and timely. In the example above, Goal No. 1 works because it is: specific (walking), measurable (3 miles), attainable (walking is easy), realistic (it's springtime and getting warmer outside), and timely (can be done before work). Goal No. 3 works because it is: specific (an affirmation), measurable (I either say it or I don't), attainable (can be done anytime and anywhere), realistic (I can recite

---

Not-So-Smart Goals

If the goals you set don't fit the SMART acronym, they aren't going to work. For example, setting the goal "I want to be happy" doesn't work because it's impossible to concretely measure happiness. Saying "I'm going to eat healthy" doesn't work if you don't define what you mean by "healthy"—it's not specific. Saying you're going to start exercising next week doesn't work because it's not measurable or specific or timely. What works are goals that are Specific, Measurable, Attainable, Realistic, and Timely—SMART.

it aloud if I'm alone or to myself when I'm dining with friends), and timely (before I begin each meal).

These sample goals are only illustrative; they are not meant to be emulated. SMART goals are intended to be highly personal and should be considered in the context of your own life and your own vulnerabilities around food and exercise. Think back to the Dear Self Letters you wrote in Step 1. It's where you want your life to be. The SMART goals you set are the rungs on that ladder to success.

When you set your SMART goals, they should always feel empowering. If not, you're going about it the wrong way. Start out by setting at least two but no more than three goals. They can be the same for every day of the week, or one or all can change daily. Do not plan out for more than a week. At the very most, you should revisit them every seventh day.

At first, I'd like you to write down your goals every day (or every day they change) and put them someplace where you can see them—in your journal, on your smartphone or tablet, or as a screen saver on your computer. As you write them, double check to make sure they are SMART. Then repeat them aloud to yourself—for example, while getting dressed in the morning or taking a shower—to reinforce how important they are to you. Hearing yourself speak them and keeping them in the forefront of your mind will help you continue to be accountable to them.

As you advance on your way to Healthy Obsession, they will become second nature to you, and you'll be able to plan them in your head. But for now, to help get you started, here's how to set them up to guarantee that they are SMART.

Specific. It's all about the details. It's not "I'm going to start jogging" or "I'm going to make sure to walk a lot." It's "I'm going to walk 3 miles three times this week." It's not "I'm going to eat healthier every day." It's "I'm going to eat five servings of vegetables and two pieces of fruit every day."

Measurable. Saying you want to walk 3 miles is measurable. So is repeating an affirmation and planning to eat fish for dinner. Check "I did it!" Or not.

Attainable. Saying you want to run a marathon in 6 months may be attainable for some people, but is it for you? If you aren't currently putting in good mileage, chances are this really isn't attainable. Challenge yourself, but stay within reach. For you, this might mean aiming to run a 5K.

Realistic. Is it realistic to say you're going to walk every single day? Maybe not, if daily exercise is new to you. Same goes for vowing to do it on Mondays, Wednesdays, and Fridays. If something comes up on Wednesday that makes it impossible for you to get out and exercise, then you fail. If you aim to go three times a week, and go Thursday instead of Wednesday, then you don't fail. Be flexible in your planning.

Timely. That means setting a limit. It's what you want to achieve today or every day this week or three times this week. It is *not* what you will do every day until you lose 30 pounds. Remember, it's the incremental goals that make it happen, and that's what makes it timely.

Now, let's give it a try. Write two or three goals you'd like to achieve in the immediate future that will help you achieve your personal mission. You can use the space below or download the document called "My Goals" from my Web site, www.elizakingsford.com, for your notebook or journal.

1. _____

2. _____

3. _____

Now you're halfway there! The only thing more important than setting daily goals is knowing if you're achieving them. At the end of each day, take a few minutes to check in with yourself and do this exercise. You can find the worksheet called "Tracking My Goals" for your notebook on my Web site or start your own in your journal. It should look like this:

Date: _____

What were my goals today?

_____

_____

_____

Did I achieve all of them? Yes _____ No _____

If not, which ones did I not achieve?

_____

_____

_____

What could I have done differently that would have changed the outcome?

_____

_____

_____

Did I overachieve any? Yes _____ No _____

If you're on track, congratulations! Give yourself a well-deserved pat on the back. You're definitely on your way to Healthy Obsession. If you fail to achieve all of your goals once in a while, say a few times a month or once a week, then you're still doing really well. Your goal is intended to show your progress, not perfection. However, if you're consistently missing your goals a few days a week, you need to revisit them. Perhaps you're overshooting their attainability. Are you being realistic? Are you not giving it your best? Are you engaging in the behaviors that will get you to achieve your goals?

Track, Track, Track

Your daily goals are *your* goals—the way you best see yourself losing weight, becoming more active, and adopting a healthy lifestyle. What's most relevant to keeping you on track? Here are some things to consider:

- Mindfulness exercises to keep you focused on the here and now
- The Dealing Skills you're practicing to break down the barriers that test your vulnerabilities
- Recording what you eat as soon as you eat it
- Planning your meals and going to the market to stock up on what you need
- Using an app or Web site to help with your meal planning
- Deciding the night before what you will eat tomorrow
- Knowing what your next meal is going to be and where it is going to come from, so you are never caught off guard
- Figuring out how you're going to build 10,000 steps into each day
- Strategizing your behaviors and choices in special situations
- Making a plan for getting back on plan if you falter

Asking yourself these questions will allow you to examine the barriers to your success.

It is not enough to change your goals; you must examine them first. What was getting in your way? What can you do differently? How can you set yourself up for success going forward?

Conversely, if you notice you are overachieving your goals on a regular basis, say more than three times in a row, it's a sign that your goals are getting too easy. Ratchet them up and make them more challenging.

THE POWER OF PLANNING

How many times have you been in this scenario?

> **Him/her:** Where do you want to go for dinner?
>
> **You:** I don't care, where do you want to go?
>
> **Him/her:** I'll go wherever you want to go.
>
> **You:** Really, I don't care. You pick.
>
> **Him/her:** You sure?
>
> **You:** Sure, I'm sure.

And before you know it, you're somewhere you really don't want to be, surrounded by people eating buckets of chicken wings. There is *nothing* on the menu that remotely fits your plan to eat fish. And you have no Plan B.

This is a perfect example of living in big-picture thinking. It is so easy to get lost. In the big-picture plan, you're stuck saying to yourself, "Oh, well, I'm here now," so you ask your friend, "What kind of wings do you want?" It's a precarious situation because you're not only annoyed with yourself for going off plan, you're also on the cusp of reverting to black-and-white thinking—"My diet's ruined, so why not order some french fries, too?"—or labeling—"I'm such a loser."

Here's the thing about SMART goals and why they're most important. In order to achieve them, you must have a plan, which brings me to Brain-Powered Pointer No. 25:

> Fail to plan, plan to fail.

If you had had a goal for the day and a plan to carry it through, like the one in the earlier example, the previous scenario would have gone like this:

> **Him/her:** Where do you want to go for dinner?
>
> **You:** I made reservations at that new fish house. Heard it's pretty good.

That's how it works when you have a plan. Planning is arguably *the* most important skill for long-term success. When you have a plan, you will rarely get into untenable situations that put you in jeopardy. It's another example proving that weight loss is not about willpower, which is counterproductive thinking because it suggests constant struggle. Weight loss is about brainpower or, more specifically in this case, SMART power. You're not struggling because you're in control.

Required Class
Give Yourself a Pep Talk

Just don't feel like it today? We all feel that way from time to time, but people with Healthy Obsession find ways to stick to their goals when "I don't feel like it" pops into their brains. Like them, get that Wise Mind working and give yourself a pep talk. Use your best persuasive powers to motivate, encourage, cajole, support, cheer, and challenge yourself. Turn it into an affirmation that will work for you. Here's the one I use: "I may not feel like it now, but I know I'm going to feel great after I've finished." Now write your own, here or in your journal:

_____

_____

_____

_____

_____

_____

_____

Without a plan, we must rely on our own instincts and our willpower, and that can make a situation really hard—"I'm surrounded by nothing but chicken wings, which I absolutely love." And that makes lapsing pretty easy.

As you now know, what we think tends to become our reality. So if we plan and keep our goals in our conscious awareness, we are more likely to make decisions in line with that goal—"I don't want to eat chicken wings; let's go someplace else"—rather than if we leave our decision making to the last minute. Having a framework to work off of in all situations makes the chances of follow-through significantly higher.

SETTING BOUNDARIES FOR YOURSELF

It's an old cliché but nevertheless so true: Life doesn't always go as planned. Neither do daily routines. There will be times when the details of a situation you're about to step into seem murky, making it feel like sticking to your goal is going to be impossible. But it's not. These are the times you need more than a map and a plan. You need boundaries to help you stay on course. Think of it this way: You accidentally make a wrong turn on your cross-country journey, and your GPS tells you to recalculate and get back on track. Would you just ignore it, keep going, and hope for the best? Or would you immediately recalculate so you can get back on the right road again without losing much ground? When you have boundaries—the wills and won'ts of your life—you instinctually know what to do.

Planning sounds very black and white when it actually needs to be gray. When the unexpected happens, you need to be flexible, but within reason. When you live with your own set of boundaries, you'll always have a backup plan—your Plan B—to smooth out the bumps in the road that are part of everyday life. As an example, let's go back to the chicken wing dilemma. The black-and-white thinking mind has you digging into the wings along with everyone else. But the boundaries you've set for yourself are there to help you override this awkward situation: You know you won't eat anything deep-fried, so you minimize the situation by ordering a grilled chicken sandwich.

Here are examples of other situations where having personal boundaries makes sticking to your goals easier. The reception area of your office tempts you every day with a big bowl of jelly beans: "I will use the side door to avoid the temptation." You arrive home and find there is nothing in the refrigerator you can eat: "I will do meal plans and food shop every Sunday." You want to go to the gym after work, but frequently find yourself too hungry: "I will eat a light snack mid-afternoon on gym days." Your office cafeteria is too tempting: "I will bring my own lunch to work and eat in the conference room." You find yourself at a restaurant where there is nothing healthy on the menu: "I will always check menus online before deciding on a restaurant." You know being home alone with nothing to do sends you to the refrigerator for idle eating: "I will always plan my downtime."

There are lots of little situations that are part of everyday life that challenge your goals. Think of your own life and come up with a list of Wills and Won'ts you want to live by. Write them down here or download the worksheet called "My Wills and Won'ts" from my Web site, www.elizakingsford.com, for your journal or notebook.

WILLS	WON'TS
1.	1.
2.	2.
3.	3.
4.	4.
5.	5.

Personal boundaries exist to help you move more fluidly from one goal to the next, from one day to the next. They help you stay mindful and live in the moment—"I won't eat at fast-food places." "I will make sure I walk every day." "I won't travel without carrying emergency snacks." They are there to help you live with intention, to keep your focus. They get you through the little bumps in life, the everyday annoyances that can get in your way. However, there are times when the road will get really rocky and you'll need stronger artillery to emerge the winner, or at least unscathed. I call this strategy "Prevent a Lapse from Becoming a Relapse," and it's where I'm taking you next.

MASTER OF WEIGHT LOSS: Mark M.

"I Couldn't Admit How Much I Ate"

I'm the first to admit that I was a reluctant "patient" when I first went to Eliza Kingsford for help. I was 150 pounds overweight, so I knew I needed help and needed it badly. Heck, I needed to lose more weight than my three kids put together. My energy, my mood, and my family life were suffering. I was not taking care of myself, but I was so overweight that I thought it was impossible. I thought I was at the point of no return.

My family was really on me about losing weight, and the end result was for me to seek counseling from Eliza. I immediately started out on the offensive: "Just tell me what you want me to eat and what I'm supposed to do to work out, and I'll do it." She patiently told me that she could help me but that first she wanted to see what I was eating. She found an app on my phone for me and told me to record everything I ate for a week. For the next 3 weeks, I sat before her with nothing to show. I just couldn't do it. I couldn't admit how much I ate. And that included to myself. I remember her saying, "Why are you hiding this from yourself? You can't manage what you don't monitor." Well, I couldn't argue with that! Somehow, it got me righted.

Eliza could see that my eating habits were terrible. So was my ability to move around. I had so little ambition. So we started out working on me, changing what I was eating and examining why I was eating. My journey was going to be a long one, which she told me to not focus on at all. "Let's set immediate doable goals that you can measure every day," she told me. I thought it was a little nutsy at first, but it turned out to be a real turning point for me.

Each week I'd reflect on how well I did in relationship to my goals, and then we'd set new ones. Sometimes we'd go back to the same goals for the week until I felt ready to move on. Setting small, immediate goals helped me realize that change was possible. Breaking down where I needed to take my life and seeing it happen one small goal at a time gave me confidence that I could achieve what I thought would never be achievable. It all started with the accountability of owning up to my food intake. I have to say that seeing it written out was a real eye-opener. Nobody needs to eat that much! I now realize that there was a whole lot more going on in my life—my mind, really—that was driving my food choices.

I'd say, right now, my biggest achievement was getting my eating under control. I only eat when I'm feeling the need for food, not the need for something else. I'm amazed at how much less I am eating than I was 6 months ago. I still have a long way to go, but I'm down 50 pounds—that's the equivalent of one of my kids. I'm not going to say it's easy because it isn't, but I can say that *understanding* what drives unhealthy eating habits is a life changer, and I plan to take it all the way. I feel so much better I can't imagine ever going backward.

Prevent a Lapse from Becoming a Relapse

Nobody is immune to food cravings, temptations, or even an all-out binge. There are physical cravings, like the ones you get from eating the addictive foods you learned about in Step 6. Then there are cravings we get for psychological reasons, the ones that are emotionally charged.

When these psychological cravings erupt, it's like your Emotional Mind is on full throttle and your Wise Mind is asleep in the backseat. If the Wise Mind was paying attention, however, it would tell you this: "You ate a doughnut— so what? Now, get back on track and move on. It was just a lapse, a little slip, a single moment in time when you deviated from your eating plan and your goals." No harm, no foul—that is, as long as that one lapse doesn't lead to another, then another, as you continue to repeat the behavior until, "Yikes, I ate four doughnuts!" And that brings me to Brain-Powered Pointer No. 26:

> **A lapse is not a problem as long as
> it does not lead to a relapse.**

I want to lay to rest one common misconception that throws so many people trying to lose weight into a full-blown "I blew it all!" panic after eating something off plan. You did not blow it all. One errant slip, even a big one— four doughnuts, an all-you-can-eat buffet in which you really got your money's worth, winning a chicken wing–eating contest—will not overnight undo 6 months or even 2 weeks of weight-loss success. A slip only becomes a problem when you allow the behavior to continue. It can trigger what I call the "what the heck" response: "That fantastic six-course dinner really hit the spot, but I really blew my plan. So, what the heck, I'll eat whatever I want for the rest of the weekend and get back on plan on Monday." Only by Monday that one indiscretion may have added up to three or four more "fantastic" meals, adding up to a whole lot of extra calories that most surely will show up on the scale. In the end, the only thing that is going to wreck your healthy eating and exercise goals is *you*—the way you respond to your errant eating and what you do next.

The way to avoid risking a relapse is to recover *now*. Not tomorrow, not Monday, not after the entire box of doughnuts is gone and out of sight. Now. That's what a person with a Healthy Obsession does.

The Causes Behind Overeating

The urge to overeat or binge is greater than mere hunger, especially in people who are overweight and/or have Resistant Biology. It comes on with an intensity that we often have to fight to resist. These are among the situations that can incite an increase in appetite.

- Extreme emotions, such as anger, anxiety, boredom, and grief
- Cognitive distortions
- Fatigue or not getting enough sleep
- Dieting that limits calories or particular foods or food groups
- Medical conditions such as insulin resistance and blood sugar swings
- Drinking alcohol or taking recreational drugs
- Being around highly palatable foods, such as items high in fat and/or sugar or other processed foods
- Thinking and talking about food
- Situations associated with eating, such as a long car trip or watching television
- Routines perceived as being in a rut
- High-risk situations (Step 10) and other triggers

LAPSES HAPPEN—EXPECT THEM

The biology of overweight makes it impossible for anybody to eat perfectly all the time. There are several reasons why this is. First, when it comes to food, studies show that the brains of people with Resistant Biology are wired differently than people who can easily say no to food. Brain scans on overweight people have found that just talking about food can activate the pleasure-seeking area of the brain, releasing dopamine and creating a craving for foods we typically think of as "sinful." Studies also show that the brains of obese individuals have fewer dopamine receptors than their normal-weight peers, thus creating the need for more of their favorite foods in order to create a dopamine response. For them, food is just harder to resist. You see a doughnut, you want to eat a doughnut.

Second, your vulnerability to desire the wrong kinds of food increases even more when you starve your fat cells by eating too little. Eventually, they're going to revolt and make a box of doughnuts seem absolutely irresistible. Remember that hunger hormone ghrelin that I described in Step 2? When you consistently restrict your calories, ghrelin starts to increase and flow through your body, making all of those cravings come to life. It's just one more example of why dieting is not a good idea! Also, when you start eating highly palatable foods, such as doughnuts or any processed food, it's hard to stop because the prefrontal cortex, the area of the brain that drives decision making, turns off.

Lastly, no one can escape our modern food culture, which intentionally entices us to overeat. You'll never find people bingeing on bags of carrots or containers of bean sprouts. When we have a bad day at the office, we want to dig our hands into the cookie jar. Marketers play right into our addiction to high-fat and sugary processed foods with this dirty little trick: They know exactly how much fat and/or sugar to put into products that will get us to reach for more and more.

For people with a weight problem, a rendezvous with the cookie jar has potentially risky consequences. If you've spent years or even decades guiding your eating habits with cognitive distortions, a single cookie can lead to a fistful—"Oops, well, I'll make up for it by skipping lunch"—which can lead to emptying the entire jar. Then that little voice starts berating, "I really blew it now, so I might as well go to lunch. I'll save my plan to eat a turkey wrap for another day when I'm eating on plan. But now, give me a bacon cheeseburger." It's like your brain hit the default button and you're back to all your old thinking errors that produce unwanted behaviors. These behaviors heighten the risk of setting off an out-of-control eating frenzy that lasts all day or all weekend, producing guilt, shame, or self-loathing for so blatantly deviating from your plan and not exerting more self-control.

Relapses often occur as a result of black-and-white thinking—the "I blew it" self-flogging that escalates when you crawl into bed with a belly too full, and the "I-ruined-it-all" fear that sets in over what the scale is going to tell you in the morning. Negative mental chatter goes into overdrive.

Hunger and food cravings are a way of life for all of us. Knowing how to respond to them in a calm, affirmative way is the bedrock to navigating the inevitable slip successfully. There are tactics you can enlist to control a food craving. And should you slip, there are ways to keep the lapse from becoming a relapse. Let's examine them all.

HOW TO MANAGE A CRAVING

Most people think that a craving is something they can't control. They believe it will just keep on nagging them until they give in. Not so. Cravings are a lot like an ocean tide: They come and go, they ebb and flow. They can rise with an incredible force, but if you're able to wait it out, they will eventually subside.

Cravings can be both psychological and physiological, but they share one commonality: You never crave cookies because your body *needs* sugar and flour. Your cravings for pizza, crackers, chocolate, and other highly palatable foods are a mixture of your brain chemistry and your psychological attachment to the food. If you are mentally able to refocus—say, by eating something healthy and on your plan, or focusing your mind on a challenging task—the craving will go away. The more you can refocus and move through the craving, the more infrequent your cravings will become. By the same token, the more you give in to a craving, the more frequently others will arise. Continually giving in reduces your ability to move through it, increasing the risk that they will become habitual.

Even though a trigger can activate your tastebuds in a nanosecond—"What's the boardwalk without cotton candy!"—the secret to not caving to a craving is to respond just as fast, which brings me to Brain-Powered Pointer No. 27:

The most effective technique to stop a craving is urge surfing.

Urge surfing is a lot like riding the waves on a surfboard, only you're doing it in your head. As a wave (your craving) builds, it comes on strong, then it subsides as it gets close to the shore. Then another wave approaches, coming on strong again, then it moves on to the shore. The idea of this technique is to surf the urge rather than fight it. Just let it come, then ride it until it subsides.

When I explain urge surfing to people, I often use chain-smokers on an overseas flight as an analogy. They know they can't smoke, but they somehow make it through 8 hours or more without a cigarette. They may not realize it, but the reason they are able to resist smoking is because they urge surf their way across the ocean.

You, too, can urge surf a craving away. The only difference between you and the overseas flier is that he is forced to urge surf; he has no choice. You, on the other hand, have to do it intentionally. It serves no purpose to try to judge the urge—"This lousy beach weather is making me crave an ice cream sundae." The key is to make a decision—"Should I or shouldn't I?"—with intention. Every single time you feel a craving coming on, turn to this exercise. The more you practice it, the more successful you'll be at it, and your cravings will become few and far between. First, I'll start with an example to help guide you.

Slow down what you are doing at the moment and think about what you are craving. "I notice I'm craving a chocolate sundae." This brings your craving to your conscious awareness.

Nonjudgmentally, observe the urge and rate how strong it is on a scale of 1 to 10 (10 being the strongest). Where might you feel it in your body? What sensations are coming up for you? "I notice I'm craving a chocolate sundae, and I feel it at about an 8. I feel some tightening in my chest and my stomach is suddenly growling." The number notifies you that you are feeling the urge pretty intensely, but you are also not attaching a judgment to the urge, good or bad. It's just there. You're just noticing it's present. Giving it your time and attention makes you pause and gives you the time to mentally move on.

Sit with the urge for a moment, if you can. Be curious about it. If you give in to this craving, how is it going to make you feel? How would surfing the urge instead make you feel? "I'm not hungry really, but I just want that ice cream. I need comfort food—fat and sugar. But I know that after I eat it, I'll feel bloated and crappy and will totally be mad at myself. If I don't give in, I'm pretty sure I'd survive. I also think I might feel empowered by being able to say no to something that won't serve me." Recognizing the repercussions

Take Binge Eating Disorder Seriously

A binge means to engage in something to excess, in this case eating. The bingeing I refer to in this book is the type that occurs intermittently, not the kind that is indicative of an eating disorder. However, there is a difference between overeating, the occasional binge, and the condition known as binge eating disorder (BED).

BED is a medical condition that needs to be treated by a health care professional and should be taken seriously. Although not all the causes of BED are known, research suggests that a chemical imbalance in the brain, family history, and traumatic life events may play a role.

BED is medically defined as the following:

- Routinely eating far more than most adults would eat at a typical meal, during a specific period of time (2 hours or less), or under specific circumstances

- Bingeing episodes that include three of the following:

    Feeling a lack of control over eating while engaging in the binge

    Eating beyond the feeling of fullness

    Overeating when not hungry

    Eating in secret to hide how much you eat

    Feeling intense shame or guilt after bingeing

- Bingeing, on average, at least once a week for 3 months

- Not trying to compensate for bingeing with extreme behavior, such as self-induced vomiting or overexercise before giving in is often a deterrent in itself. And feeling powerful when you don't give in to something that is not serving you can feel pretty good, too. Sit with the urge as long as you feel comfortable doing so.

Make a choice. The decision is yours—"I'm going to take a bike ride. I think it will make me feel so good that I won't want to spoil it by eating something filling and fattening like a sundae." Do not judge your decision either way.

The more you practice this technique, the easier it will become to surf your urges. At first, you may find that you give in to more cravings than you'd like. However, if you stick with it and repeatedly practice, I promise it will get easier.

Now, it's your turn to give it a try. Remember to go through this exercise every single time you feel a craving coming on. You can practice here or download the document called "Urge Surfing" from my Web site, www.elizakingsford.com, for your journal or notebook.

Slow down what you are doing at the moment and think about what you are craving. What is it?

_____

_____

Nonjudgmentally, observe the urge and rate how strong it is on a scale of 1 to 10 (10 being the strongest). Where might you feel it in your body? What sensations are coming up for you?

_____

_____

_____

_____

Sit with the urge for a moment, if you can. Be curious about it. If you give in to this craving, how is it going to make you feel? How would surfing the urge instead make you feel?

_____

_____

_____

_____

Make a choice:

_____

_____

_____

_____

In addition to urge surfing, you can also enlist these tactics:

Distract yourself. You're on the boardwalk, and it seems like every other vendor is selling french fries. The smell alone is making your mouth water; you want some so much. Rather than give in, distract yourself in some notable way—"Let's go on the Ferris wheel!"—and the craving will disappear. Leave the room, leave the building, or whatever it takes to get out of the target zone of what may be tempting you.

Think about your quest for Healthy Obsession. People with a Healthy Obsession get cravings, too, but not in the way an overweight person does. As I've already noted, as you continue on your journey to Healthy Obsession by getting away from processed, fatty, and sugary foods, your cravings for them will gradually diminish, though they will probably never totally go away. Ask yourself, "How will eating this food serve me? What is the benefit to eating it?" The obvious answer is eating the food won't serve you and there is no physical benefit to eating it. To someone with a Healthy Obsession, this is usually enough to walk away from it.

Carry a safety snack. This is what someone with Healthy Obsession will always do. When a craving hits, eating something can work to decrease the craving, especially if it comes on when you're hungry. It's the reason I always have a safety snack nearby—in my desk, car, and handbag—and I never travel without them. My safety snacks include foods such as nuts, pretzels, and some cheese to eat with fruit. Remember to be careful and read labels when buying your safety snacks. You want to make sure you buy items without mystery ingredients and with little to no added sugars.

STOP A CRAVING FROM BECOMING A BINGE

Bingeing doesn't happen in a haphazard way. There is a lot of distorted thinking going on in your brain before you stick a fork into an entire double chocolate layer cake. I talk to clients about bingeing all the time, and each time I ask what happened, I get a response that goes something like this: "I don't know, it just happened. I just suddenly found myself raiding the refrigerator."

You know by now that binges don't "just happen," even though that's the way they can feel. Acting out a different outcome allows you to learn from the experience. By mentally walking through preferred alternatives to bingeing and visualizing how to act differently, you can help better your chances of a different outcome going forward. So, get in your Wise Mind and let's examine your history of overeating and bingeing. You can do this in the space provided here or download the document called "My Overeating History" from my Web site, www.elizakingsford.com, for your notebook or journal.

Think of three different times you can remember really well when you binged or overate.

1. _____

2. _____

3. _____

For each situation, answer the following:

Situation 1

What happened? Be as specific as possible.

_____
_____
_____
_____

What people, places, things, and feelings contributed to this?

_____
_____
_____
_____

Looking back, what—if anything—could you have done differently to avoid the binge trigger?

_____
_____
_____
_____

Looking back, what could you have done differently to minimize the damage it caused your goals and plan?

_____

_____

_____

_____

If you had the opportunity to relive this situation, what would you do differently?

_____

_____

_____

_____

Situation 2

What happened? Be as specific as possible.

_____

_____

_____

_____

What people, places, things, and feelings contributed to this?

_____

_____

_____

_____

Looking back, what—if anything—could you have done differently to avoid the binge trigger?

_____

_____

_____

_____

Looking back, what could you have done differently to minimize the damage it caused your goals and plan?

_____

_____

_____

_____

If you had the opportunity to relive this situation, what would you do differently?

_____

_____

_____

_____

Situation 3

What happened? Be as specific as possible.

_____

_____

_____

_____

What people, places, things, and feelings contributed to this?

_____

_____

_____

_____

Looking back, what—if anything—could you have done differently to avoid the binge trigger?

_____

_____

_____

_____

Looking back, what could you have done differently to minimize the damage it caused your goals and plan?

_____

_____

_____

_____

If you had the opportunity to relive this situation, what would you do differently?

_____

_____

_____

_____

Now, let's practice some binge control. Promise yourself that before you give in to out-of-control eating, you will look at the situation from all perspectives and identify all possible outcomes, a technique I call Pro/Con Chatter. The choice is yours to make. You don't have to give in to the binge, and maybe you won't if you allow yourself the time to consider the consequences. I always tell people, if the consequences are okay with you, then go ahead and eat off plan. They almost never do.

Here is an example of the Pro/Con exercise:

I have an urge to: Eat Oreo cookies.

What is causing this urge? I've been craving them. I saw an ad for Oreos, and I can't stop thinking about how they would taste.

What are the pros of giving in to this urge?

1. It will satisfy my craving.
2. I will really enjoy the taste.
3. I haven't had an Oreo in at least a year.
4. I've been really good about my eating and feel like I deserve a treat.

What are the cons of giving in to this urge?

1. I have to go buy them and then the bag will be in my pantry, which means at some point I'll eat the entire bag.
2. I probably won't be able to stop at just one cookie.
3. Oreos don't offer any nutrients.
4. Oreos are filled with sugar, and sugar is a trigger for me, which will probably cause me to eat more of the things I'm choosing not to eat.

Next time you have the urge to overeat or feel a binge coming on, turn to this exercise, or download several of the documents called "Pro/Con Chatter" from my Web site, www.elizakingsford.com, and put them in your journal.

I have an urge to:

_____

_____

What is causing this urge?

_____

_____

What are the pros of giving in to this urge? (list them all):

1. _____
2. _____
3. _____
4. _____

What are the cons of giving in to this urge?

1. _____
2. _____
3. _____
4. _____

THE ART OF HARM REDUCTION

While ideally you'd love to follow your eating and exercise plan to a tee day in and day out, you're going to find that it is virtually impossible. There will be occasions that will tempt you to eat off plan on a regular basis, perhaps even daily. Sometimes you'll even find yourself in situations where off plan is your *only* choice. It happens to people with a Healthy Obsession all the time, only they know how to work their way around it.

Let's say your spouse gets a big promotion, and the new boss is taking you out to celebrate at his favorite restaurant—a Texas barbecue joint where chicken-fried steak is the signature dish. He bellows, "Chicken-fried all around!" You may be screaming to yourself, "All I want is a salad and grilled chicken," but you want to be politically correct for your spouse's sake, so you reluctantly smile without protest, while wondering to yourself, "How can I get through all this without too much damage?" You do it by employing a technique called harm reduction, a psychological approach that is most often used for people who are unwilling or unable to stop substance abuse. Its focus is on preventing harm—in this case, eating in a restaurant practically oozing with fatty and greasy foods because you can't beg off the invitation. And that brings me to Brain-Powered Pointer No. 28:

> Harm reduction is a tactic important
> to your long-term success.

Practicing harm reduction allows you to minimize the damage in a situation in which staying on plan at the moment is looking pretty bleak. At times when a slip seems inevitable, this strategy most assuredly can keep the damage to your plan to a minimum and prevent the slip from turning into an all-out binge or a relapse. This is the same technique I teach to help people recover from a binge.

For some people, practicing harm reduction is almost a way of life, especially for folks who live in areas of the country or in households where healthy eating is not the culture. I use it all the time, as do people with a Healthy Obsession. Here is how you practice harm reduction.

Think strategically. When faced with unhealthy choices, think in terms of what you can do rather than what you don't want to do. For example, you can tell the waiter to either hold the gravy on your order or put it on the side and then ignore it. While you're at it, you can ask him to hold the french fries, too. A plain baked potato, or even no potato at all, is a better choice. When the dish is served, you can cut the meat in half, scrape off the fried breading, and ignore the other half. Order a salad, dressing on the side, and eat it before you approach the entrée, to help fill you up. Situations like this always call for using your imagination. Reduce the harm as far as you can take it.

Don't count calories. Sometimes seeing the exact number of calories on your plate can lead you to eat even more ("Holy cow! The chicken-fried dinner he just ordered must be close to a thousand calories!"). That's frightening, especially since you know it's not your choice. So, you decide the best solution for tonight's indiscretion is to make up for it tomorrow by skipping a meal or cutting calories to an extreme. Don't do it! It only means you will turn eating poorly at one meal into a full day of eating off plan and risking the hunger pangs that will go with it. Hunger pangs can be a surefire invitation to another session of overeating. Instead, affirm to get back on track at your very next meal. Write yourself an affirmation and stick it in your head: "I am going right back on plan at my very next meal." It's your surest way to minimize any damage and move forward.

Talk some sense into yourself. Black-and-white thinking is the mind-set that most often triggers a binge—"I can't believe I poured the gravy on my chicken-fried steak and ate the whole thing. Plus, I piled my potato with butter. Here comes the dessert cart. Hmm, might as well call the entire night a disaster."

Following one error with another makes absolutely no sense. Constantly remind yourself that a slip on your food plan is just that—a slip. A momentary blip that happened once in one day. Why would you want to make it two, three, or even more? When you analyze it logically, one little slip cannot ruin all the good you've done over weeks or months. Trouble only starts to brew when you let that one slip become multiple meals day after day. So, stay focused in your Wise Mind and repeat, repeat, repeat: "It's only one slip in one day. Move on."

Enlist your support system. It's rare for someone to indulge in a binge socially. It's something we almost always do when we're alone with our not-so-sensible thoughts. When the urge seems irresistible, seek out a friend or

Coping versus Lapsing

Lapsing can create a vicious cycle, as illustrated here. Coping produces a very different outcome. Coping techniques will prevent a lapse from becoming a relapse.

THE LAPSING CYCLE	THE COPING CYCLE
Coping strategies are ignored or not effective,	Using my Dealing Skills to prevent overeating
which leads to overeating,	means I'll prevent or limit overeating,
which causes decreased confidence—"I CAN'T control my eating"— which results in blame, self-pity, and guilt,	which increases my confidence—"I CAN control my eating"—
and results in decreased attention to eating and exercise, and increased overeating and decreased interest in exercise.	and keeps me focused on healthy eating and daily movement.

family member who knows the commitment you've made to a healthy life-style. Share your feelings with someone you trust and can help you move on. I have a friend who will text me, "I have my hand in a bag of Starburst jelly beans. HELP!" And I will call or text her back, "Tell me your goal. What are you working toward? Will the Starburst help you get there?" We work through her urge until she decides what she wants to do.

When all else fails, slip up better. Take the path of least resistance. That fried calamari sure is tempting, but asparagus tempura can satisfy the same mouthfeel and your desire for something crunchy and fried. It's not ideal, but it's the healthier choice. Always, always, always err on the side of healthy.

HOW TO BE A GOOD COPER

Any kind of emotion can cause you to overeat, even being happy. The emotions that are the toughest on us, though, are the negative ones, especially shame, anger, guilt, and anxiety. Research on behavior shows that an effective way to overcome the negative emotions that drive us to overeat is to steer your thoughts in the opposite direction.

Let's say, for example, you're home alone and miserable because it seems like everybody but you got invited to the cocktail party being given by the young couple who just moved into the incredibly awesome new house on the block. You're dying to see the house and be part of the new crowd. You've cooed over their dog every time you've walked by their house and engaged in small talk—"Hey, we should get together." But you're the only one not at the get-together. It fills you with a stream of negativity, causing you to lose your emotional composure and think in extremes: "Why doesn't anyone like me?" And you sink your spoon into a gallon of ice cream.

When you totally think with your Emotional Mind, your thoughts will be distorted and so will your actions—you'll overeat or binge. You have to get back into your Wise Mind, so you can think and act rationally. One way you can do this is to nudge your brain into the opposite direction.

Acting out a positive or desired behavior when you're in an opposite frame of mind is an acquired skill. It starts with keeping Brain-Powered Pointer No. 29 foremost in your mind:

The present moment is the only one I can control.

This is your number one coping skill because it is the only thing you can control, especially during times of disappointment and other stressful occurrences that make it feel like your world is spinning out of control. Does not being invited to one party mean that *nobody* likes you? Of course not. And turning to unhealthy behaviors isn't going to hurt anyone but yourself, so why are you doing it?

Navigating situations that may bring on a lapse or binge can only occur when you're in your Wise Mind. It's how you become a good coper and overcome the situations that challenge your goals. It begins with starting to calm yourself down by taking a slow, deep breath, mindfully focusing on your number one coping skill: "The present moment is the only one I can control. I will choose something that will work FOR me and not AGAINST me."

When you believe in your own capacity to cope, it fortifies your self-esteem and your ability to say no to food in times of temptation and struggle. Being a good coper enables you to:

Acknowledge your own emotional pressure points of vulnerability. "Every time I see my mother-in-law, she starts nitpicking me about something I do or wear." Keep a measure of emotional composure—"When she starts in on me, I'll make an excuse to leave."

Consider the consequences of a situation and act according to your best judgment. "Every time she does this to me, I go home angry and hit the fridge." Not anymore. You've learned to get out of the car and take a long walk until you've cooled down.

Be up-front about exactly what is bothering you. For example, rather than getting all bent out of shape when you walk into your in-laws' house, imagine how much calmer you'd be if you let your in-laws or your spouse know what's bothering you and request that it stop.

Be as realistic as possible about a situation. Prevent yourself from blowing it out of proportion. For example, when your mother-in-law says, "Oh, my, look at that dress on you," what makes you think it's a jab? It could be a compliment.

Consider intermediate steps you can take that will steer you to the best outcome. For example, you can examine the situation and chain back to figure out what led up to an eating episode. Identify the links you can break and then next time, break them. For example, if your mother-in-law only starts picking on you when you visit alone, then only go to her house if your spouse or one of your kids is with you.

Avoid thinking in extremes that tend to warp good judgment. Instead of thinking, "Damn, I just wish she'd get out of my life," be less extreme and acknowledge, "Wow, this is a really difficult relationship for me. I wish things were different."

Restrain from making imaginary or idealized wishes in favor of practical and attainable goals. For example, instead of wishing your mother-in-law out of your life, you could think, "I really should make an effort to get to know her better."

Recognize that there are a number of choices beyond black-and-white thinking. Not every visit with your mother-in-law turns out unpleasant. But your frustration with her does not have to end with you eating three extra slices of pizza. You have a lot of choices you could make that won't make you feel worse in the end.

Avoid self-pity, bitterness, and unwarranted pessimism or optimism—"She hates me"—and use denial as a temporary distraction. For example,

---

Mental Resilience Technique: Regroup

You have just "blown it" (your words) at Friday night happy hour, and you are tempted to let it ride for the rest of the weekend. You say to yourself, "How could I have been so careless? I was doing so well." When you think this way, yes, you really *have* blown it. Instead, reinforce with this mental resilience exercise:

STOP. Whatever maladaptive choice you are considering, immediately come to a halt in your thinking and actions.

AFFIRM. State an affirmation immediately: "What's done is done. It's okay to let it go and move on. My next decision will be one in line with my goals."

REPEAT. Say it again. And then say it some more 10 minutes later and 20 minutes after that. Keep going until you get yourself righted.

Even if you don't believe the affirmation in the moment, it's important you still say it. Saying it out loud is best. Saying it while standing in front of a mirror is even better. This exercise *works*. There are thousands of Long-Term Weight Controllers who can attest to it.

if you can't get her to stop judging your choice in clothing, maybe just for today you can decide it doesn't bother you. Pretend you didn't hear it and move on.

Monitor and correct your own behaviors around food and seek guidance when needed. "I recognize that I'm only reaching for this ice cream because I'm frustrated, I think I'll talk to my husband about what's bothering me instead."

Use your best Dealing Skills. It is the best artillery for overcoming untenable situations.

ACCEPT AND FORGIVE YOURSELF

Getting annoyed and angry with yourself for making a slip is risky business. It puts you on a negative path in which one slip can lead to another, then another, until you can't seem to stop yourself. Each transgression will make you feel bad and make your behavior worse, which will only make you angrier.

By now you know there's no point in that. Instead, turn off that nagging voice in your head and think back to all you learned about mindfulness in Step 4 and forgive yourself your transgression: "It's done, it's over, now move on." Repeat this affirmation, "I am a healthy person, and I desire to recommit." The quicker you respond with positive self-talk following an eating slip, the quicker you'll recover.

Think back to your past binges and times when you overate. Recall how it physically made you feel afterward: bloated, sluggish, heavy, and unhappy with yourself for going off plan; and frustrated that you're engaging in the same old behaviors that have gotten you somewhere you don't want to be. Recognizing how much you *don't* want to revisit this in itself can be a deterrent. You can also use one or all of the following tactics.

Press the pause button. Slow yourself down and re-center. This book, and Step 4 in particular, are peppered with mindfulness practices designed to draw you back into the present moment. Here are a few more:

- Write yourself a list of all the worries and distresses that are crowding your mind and clamoring for attention. Then burn the list or tuck it in your wallet for later attention.

- Focus on something pleasant and beautiful in your immediate environment—a painting, a color, a flower, a blade of grass. Allow the beauty to slow your mind. Focus; take slow, controlled breaths.

- Close your eyes and take a deep breath. Visualize yourself being transported to something you love—a sunrise or sunset, a beach with the waves lapping the water's edge, a favorite vacation spot.

- Relax your chest muscles and open up your breathing with a vigorous massage along the midline and across the chest below your collarbone.

Search for your point of vulnerability. Every time you overeat or binge, every time you lapse, and every time you relapse, it is preceded by a situation and thought process that triggered the emotion that turned you to food. You learned this in Step 3. Use the Chaining technique you learned on page 50 and go back and identify the chain of events that led to your lapse or binge. Only through being aware of your points of vulnerability will you be able to avoid them or plan for them going forward.

Recognize it's not about the food. Your mouth may be watering for a foot-long ham hoagie, but here's the reality: Typically, if you are a healthy eater, you should be able to fulfill that taste craving after the first two or three bites, as pleasure-centered dopamine is released. Once dopamine is released, continuing to indulge the craving is just habitual or psychological eating. However, if you're addicted to highly palatable processed, sugary, and/or fatty foods, it is going to take more bites to get the urge to subside. By the time you finish the last bite of the foot-long, dig into the potato chips, and then something else, the reason you are eating is no longer about the food. It's all about your behaviors and the messages your brain is sending you.

Here's the honest truth: If you truly are craving a ham hoagie, you'll enjoy it much more if you only eat a piece of it and give the rest away. And it goes without saying that you'll feel better about yourself, too. Eating mindfully, as described on page 63, can make it happen. When you have the ability to take a little to satisfy a craving and leave the rest, you'll feel proud and empowered.

Don't let a craving replace your need for something healthy. If you are physically hungry, ranch Dorito chips and potato salad are not what your body is asking for. That's your psyche talking. A hungry body wants something nourishing to keep your organs in top performance. If you're going to dip into the Doritos, honor your psyche's hunger by eating two or three, then move on to a nourishing meal. Not only are you doing your body good, but you are preventing yourself from the emotional letdown you'll feel as a result of indulging in an unhealthy eating behavior.

Say something kind to yourself. Berating yourself and beating yourself up over the three margaritas and the basket of chips you just devoured will only make the situation worse. As you've already learned, those messages send you into the Lethargy Cycle of Self-Defeating Thoughts you learned about on page 69. Avoid this by stopping your behavior and saying something kind to yourself right away. Even if you don't believe it in your moment of self-annoyance, you'll come around to believing it faster than you think. Here are examples of personal to-yourself affirmations that can help get you back on track:

"My food choices don't define who I am."

"I have the power to change my course whenever I choose."

"I will not be unkind to myself for making this decision. It doesn't help me get to where I want to be."

Becoming a Long-Term Weight Controller is all about mental preparedness. In the next chapter, I'm going to show you how to navigate high-risk situations, the land mines that make a slip feel totally out of your control.

MASTER OF WEIGHT LOSS: Amy K.

"I Was a Food Addict"

People who knew me then and now can't believe I'm the same person. That's how much changing my relationship with food has changed my life. And I am forever grateful to Eliza Kingsford for making it happen.

"Then" was about 5 years ago, when I weighed 200ish pounds—that's a lot considering I'm only 5-foot-4. "Now" is me 65 pounds lighter, looking great—if I do say so myself—and oh so healthy. And grateful, too, for what I've accomplished.

I can't believe where I was 5 years ago. I would just eat, eat, eat all the time. I didn't eat because I was hungry; I ate because it was there, or because everybody else was eating, or because it looked good. Once I started, I couldn't stop until I was overly full, sometimes almost to the point of feeling ill. I felt powerless against food. I swear I had food on my mind from the time I woke up in the morning until I went to bed at night. There were times I'd find myself in front of the fridge looking for anything I could get my hands on. I couldn't understand why, as I wasn't even hungry.

My first question after I told all this to Eliza was, "What's wrong with me? It can't be natural." She responded with questions of her own, starting with, "What is it that you like to eat? What do you find so irresistible?" I rattled off a bunch of stuff like cookies, sodas, and chips, ice cream, pizza, burgers, and fries. She looked at me knowingly, and I thought she was going to lecture me with, "There's nothing healthy about that!" Only she didn't. She told me that all the highly processed sugary foods I liked to eat had hijacked my brain. I was a food addict. I never even knew such a thing was possible. As it turned out, there was *a lot* I didn't know and understand about my relationship with food.

Eliza chained me back through my habits to help me find the triggers, both psychological and physiological, that drove me to food. I began to understand that one of my biggest triggers was my relationship with my husband. We had some marital discord that we were avoiding, and, for me, that meant numbing my frustration with food. Eliza taught me that I needed to become more aware of my triggers and play a more intentional role in my own life. She taught me how to control my emotional mind and live more in my Wise Mind, which allowed me to recognize the triggers that were leading me to food.

For me, this was a turning point. I went from thinking about food all the time to changing the way I think when I'm around food. There's a big difference between the two! Rather than eat mindlessly, I now stop and mindfully make a decision about every food choice I make. This is what helped me wean myself away from processed foods and get my food addiction under control. Being mindful also helped me face my marital problem and push for my husband and me to seek counseling.

Today, I no longer feel powerless around food. My marriage survived counseling, and I feel that I have tackled my food addiction. I still struggle with lapsing from time to time—still love chips—but I don't let it turn into a relapse. I now use my mental tools to prevent that, because I never want to go back there again. I make choices that don't cause my biology to get hijacked. I don't ever want to be in that position again. I've learned to live more in my Wise Mind and be intentional about my food choices, which got me out from under the crushing weight of my food addiction. I still have to be mindful every day about my relationship with food, as I now recognize that it's a lifelong process. And I'm fine with it because, for what feels like the first time in my life, I am in control of my life around food rather than allowing food to control my life.

Outsmart High-Risk Situations

osing weight and keeping it off could be a whole lot easier if life didn't get in the way. But it does. When vacations, celebrations, holidays, and even bad weather ("Let's have a snow party!") roll around, the mind of a weight controller cackles, "Let's eat." Then there are bad moods, bad days, disappointments, emergencies, and the no-getting-away-from-it stress that all try to talk us into putting weight loss on hold for a while ("I'd be having a whole lot more fun at this bachelor party weekend if I could eat and drink like crazy just like everybody else.").

Life happens, and when things don't go our way or feel like they're getting out of control, even briefly, the Negative Ned that's been living in your brain starts shouting so loud you'll eat anything just to shut him up—"I'll take three pulled-pork tacos and a big pint of stout!"

It happens to all of us from time to time. When I begin one-on-one counseling with clients, invariably the conversation leads to past situations that have derailed their diets: "I went on a cruise, and there was so much food." Or "We celebrated our anniversary with a six-course dinner and a bottle of champagne," followed by the panicky "I ruined everything!" Or "My mother got so sick and I just couldn't keep it together. Monitoring what I eat was THE LAST thing on my mind!" And, of course, the classic "I was doing great until the holidays came along and I gained back practically everything."

Does any of this mental chatter sound familiar? Probably so, at least on a base level. Weight loss often gets derailed because something always gets in the way, usually something unexpected that didn't fit snugly into your perfect plan for putting life on hold for a while until you could get back into that little black dress. Only now, you're finally getting it—that's not reality. There is no putting life on hold. You are *always* going to run into circumstances that test and try your resolve. You are *always* going to be watching your weight. To put new meaning to an old cliché, there's no such thing as a free lunch. Calories *always* count, and your Resistant Biology is always going to be there to catch the overflow.

A high-risk situation can be any occasion that has the ability to cause you to behave in ways that are not in line with your weight-loss goals. Encountering high-risk situations is all part of the journey because, well, life happens. Beyond the inevitable calorie-laden festivities—holidays, vacations, weekend bashes—there are the more subtle triggers that catch us unaware: arriving home from work frazzled, missing meals and suddenly feeling famished, the lure of Friday night happy hour ("You *are* coming with us, aren't you?"). And there are the situations that make our stress levels soar, which are a double whammy for your weight-loss effort because, as you learned in Step 2, the body's stress response produces hormones that make fat storage much more convenient.

Yes, stuff happens, but here's your new reality: This time, it's only going to get in the way of you and your goals *if you let it*, which brings me to Brain-Powered Pointer No. 30:

> The way to outsmart a high-risk situation is to face it with your mental machinery fully loaded.

You've already learned all the key strategies that are helping you change your mind-set from a Negative Ned, always doubting or questioning yourself, to a confident, mindful decision maker. Hopefully, you're already practicing them daily; you may already know them by rote, or at least you feel they are becoming second nature to you.

But there are always going to be those times that really put you to the test, when push comes to shoving you relentlessly. You'll never be in a more precarious position than when any combination of anticipation, celebration, excitement, stress, tension, trauma, frivolity, or obligation collide to put you face-to-face with a high-risk situation in which the reason to overindulge has your name written all over it. It's the ultimate emotional eating explosion.

AFFIRMATIVE ACTION: YOUR BEST DEFENSE

I am not going to say that you will never again get in situations in which you end up throwing all caution into the proverbial feed bucket. But as I've said, they will occur less often—even to the point where they become almost nonexistent—as you continue to get more comfortable in your mental makeover.

However, you will never totally get rid of your tendency to fall back on your destructive behaviors. The behaviors of your past are so deeply seeded they won't totally disappear and, unfortunately, they tend to want to come back when you're at your most vulnerable, when you're faced with a high-risk situation. This is why you've got to become assertive about the healthy new way you want to live your life. Being assertive really isn't so hard, but getting *comfortable* at being assertive can be difficult for a lot of people. If you have a weight problem, you are likely one of them.

By being assertive about your new lifestyle, I mean being able to advocate for yourself and your goals in any situation. Maintaining control of high-risk situations is often difficult because you get caught up in the emotions of not wanting to offend someone. You take a piece of your mother-in-law's famous Boston cream pie because you think saying "no, thank you" is being disrespectful. You order the prime rib and double-stuffed baked potato when you're out to lunch with the boss because he chided, "You're not one of those 'I'm just going to eat a salad' types, are you?" You dig into the ribs at the Fourth of July picnic because Big John spent all day smoking them, slathering them with South Carolina barbecue sauce, and is wearing a grin the size of a crescent moon when he sets the platter in front of you. Really, can you possibly refuse when he starts to slide a big bunch of them onto your plate? Well, yes you can.

There are people who can passionately plea their opinion in a meeting of colleagues, argue until they win in a spat with their spouse, or sweet-talk a police officer when they're pulled over for a speeding violation, but they can't get the right words out of their mouth when being pushed by a buddy who wants to load them up with barbecued ribs. Virtually every person I've come across in my work tells me that, when it comes to social interactions, they don't know how to be assertive about food.

Everywhere you go, you are going to come across people trying to push food on you. It is the most common risk factor all weight controllers share. Most of the time, these people are well-intentioned—friends who love to cook and feed people, relatives who say "I love you" with food, hosts who don't think you're having a good time if you're not partying hearty with plenty of food and drink. There's an emotional connection surrounding you, them, and the food. Food is a universal binder, and this makes it all the more difficult to say no.

When it comes to high-risk situations, it's often not so much the circumstance itself, but the people behind the situation who lead to breaking your will. After all, can you really say no to your boss when she hands you an eggnog at the annual holiday office party? Well, of course you can. I'm going to show you how.

A Lesson in Assertiveness

Being an assertive eater is one of the most important exercises I teach because you're going to rely on it *all the time*. It is an effective tool not just with friends and relatives who try to push food on you, but with strangers who control social situations in which you must dare to be different. It will help give you the gumption to finally tell Aunt Betsy that you're breaking tradition and having the family reunion at your house this year so you can be in control of the menu. It will help you find the tenacity to speak up to the waitperson and ask to have your meal cooked to your healthy requirements when you're out to dinner. And, it will get you to stop your children from nagging you to take the family out for ice cream each night of your beach vacation.

Assertiveness works because it breaks a link in the chain of all the triggers that put you in any variety of high-risk situations. It's just another form of the Chaining exercises you are beginning to master. Here's what you do:

Use a firm tone of voice. Tone of voice and facial expression are crucial. You must display that you are serious about your needs. Specifically, it is most helpful to use a calm, clear voice and have a neutral expression on your face to show the person that there is no doubt in your mind as to your desire: "No martini, thank you. I much prefer a diet cola." This doesn't mean you are cold or rude. It just means you aren't wavering. It stops people from asking the confidence-killing question, "Are you sure?"

Maintain eye contact. Making eye contact as you speak is equally important. If you don't look the person in the eyes, he or she will think that you are not serious about what you're saying and likely will egg you on: "Well, maybe you shouldn't, but just one pig-in-a-blanket isn't going to hurt, now will it?" So, look that host straight in the eye and give a firm, "No, thank you, those look delicious, but I am going to pass."

Be clear and unambiguous about your desires. It matters not how you say it, but what you say. Remember, the firm answer is, "No, thank you."

Not, "I don't think I want one." Not, "Maybe later" or "Not just yet." Always give an honest answer so it's clear that you are not going to eat whatever the pusher is pushing. Being tentative about whether you want the hors d'oeuvre only leaves doubt in the host's mind as to your real intentions. Similarly, if the waitperson hears, "If it's not too much bother, could you . . . ?" he might underestimate your request and not want to bother the chef. So, state clearly, "Please tell the chef I do not want my fish with butter sauce. Just grilled and plain."

Make sure to give a compliment. This is particularly important when you're in social gatherings, such as a dinner party or celebration, and you worry about offending the host. All hosts want their guests to have a good time, and seeing you eating or drinking too little relative to other revelers might give the impression that you are not having a good time. You can counteract this by making sure you gush with a compliment: "The food just looks so wonderful and smells divine. I can't tell you enough how much I'm enjoying your dinner party." It will put your host at ease about you enjoying yourself and also get him to stop running that tray of pigs-in-a-blanket under your nose.

Suggest an alternative. This may not be necessary in all situations but can be your savior in others. In some situations—family gatherings, weekends away with friends, the annual neighborhood progressive dinner—people can be relentless about wanting to feed you until they feel you are as happy and satisfied as everybody else at the party. In situations such as these, your best solution for not indulging in the foods or drinks you don't want is to suggest an alternative. Offer to bring crudités and low-fat dip for the cocktail hour. Suggest offering sorbet as an addition to the dessert menu. Bring your own nonalcoholic cocktail in a martini shaker. When people see you're serious about what you're doing, they'll generally let you be . . . as long as you are joining in on the fun, of course.

Reinforce it all with a coping statement. Think back to when you were a kid. Getting together with family and friends was *all* about the play and hardly about the food. Fun was playing ball with your cousins, swimming in the lake, or chasing lightning bugs by the campfire. Write yourself a coping statement you can relate to that emphasizes the nonfood experience of the high-risk situation you are in, such as: "Getting together with family and good friends is all about love, not about food."

Prep Think for High-Risk Scenarios

Certain events become high-risk eating situations because there is an emotional connection in your life between each circumstance and food. Think about it. If you served a chicken breast and broccoli at Thanksgiving instead of the traditional dinner with all the trimmings, you wouldn't have a nostalgic connection to the food. Maybe you'd think of it only as a time to spend with loved ones.

Take about 10 minutes to think about the high-risk situations you typically encounter. Then put pen in hand and write them in the space below or download the document "High-Risk Scenarios" from my Web site, www.elizakingsford.com, for your notebook or journal.

1. _____   6 _____

2. _____   7 _____

3. _____   8 _____

4. _____   9 _____

5. _____   10 _____

Now, for each situation, ask yourself the following first three questions. Keep in mind everything you've learned so far about yourself, your food triggers, your food history, past slips, and your ability to stick with your goals. Write down your answers. Next time one of these situations comes up, come back to this exercise and follow through with questions four and, if necessary, five. This is the exercise you'll come back to each time you are confronted with a high-risk situation. Keep at it until you get to the conclusion, "It worked bigtime!" You'll get there, I promise. Everybody always does.

The situation:

_____

_____

1. What is my history in dealing with this situation? (Pay close attention to the food patterns.)

   _____
   _____
   _____
   _____

2. What were the triggers that caused me to turn to food for comfort?

   _____
   _____
   _____
   _____

3. How can I try to do something different next time so I won't end up straying/bingeing?

   _____
   _____
   _____
   _____

4. How did it work?

   _____
   _____
   _____
   _____

5. If it didn't work as expected, ask yourself: What can I do next time to have a more positive outcome?

   _____
   _____
   _____
   _____

DEFENSIVE ACTIONS FOR POTENTIALLY DESTRUCTIVE TIMES

As individuals we're all different, and that means we all have our own personal high-risk situations that can threaten to get between us and our goals. Some of my clients report getting unrelenting cravings for certain comfort foods, such as meat loaf or chicken potpie, in the winter when the chill sets in. Others say that increased summertime social food functions—picnics, three big holidays so close together—kick in a feeding frenzy that barely stops until after Labor Day. In the meantime, the pounds add up.

One client, Denise F., told me that she looks so forward to Thanksgiving dinner at her family home 3 hours away and thinks about it so much her mouth starts watering in anticipation as soon as she crosses the border to her hometown. Crossing the threshold to her mother's house was a *huge* trigger for her. "It's family recipes I've loved since childhood, and I only get to eat them once a year," she told me, adding that she *always* overeats at the meal and relishes the leftovers for days to come. Prior to seeing me, Thanksgiving was the beginning of a holiday-long spiral that would end in a 5-to-10-pound weight gain come New Year's.

In situations like Denise's, going through the coping technique called Prep Think for High-Risk Scenarios becomes especially important. I went through the steps with Denise, telling her to ask herself: "What is *my history* with this situation? What were my triggers? What can I do differently next time? How did it go?"

In the end, it was one simple strategy that made a huge difference in how Denise approached and eventually got through the holidays. Instead of going to her mother's house for Thanksgiving dinner, she invited her family to her own home where she could control the menu and she could send the leftovers home with her relatives. "Funny how getting through that first Thanksgiving with a different venue changed everything for me," she says. "I've been doing Thanksgiving ever since, and it doesn't trigger a feeding frenzy that starts a month before Christmas. I still gain a pound or two over the holidays but *nothing* like it used to be. I don't even miss my grandmother's recipes, I think because I'm not at my mother's house where the food was for all those years. It was the sentiment, I think, more than the taste."

One pivotal change, one *huge* difference, one *major* achievement.

I point this out because, like Denise, you're going to find that making just one change can make a whole lot of difference when it comes to staying true to your goals while facing a high-risk situation. However, you're going to find yourself in a lot of circumstances in which you aren't going to have the luxury of going through Prep Think. The impromptu "Let's go out for happy hour" is a good example. Another: You spend 2 hours stuck in traffic and arrive home hungry with dinner an hour away. What do you do? You've got to plan a quick-fix coping technique, customized to what works for you.

To help you get started, this chart lists 20 common high-risk scenarios and the quick coping techniques that have helped the clients I've coached over the years. They'll work for you, too.

Potential High-Risk Event	Quick Coping Response
1. Going out to dinner	Look up the menu online and decide what you will order before you go. Do not open the menu in the restaurant. It will only tempt you to change your mind.
2. Big restaurant portions	Ask the waitperson for a to-go box when you order your meal, so that you can pack up half of it to take home before you even take your first bite. Or share an entrée with a willing friend.
3. It's cold outside and you're craving comfort food—chicken potpie, meat loaf, lasagna	Nothing says you can't have it, but you don't need to blow your calorie budget. Look for healthier versions of your comfort food favorites. As you get more accustomed to eating whole foods, you'll love healthier versions of your old favorites just as much—possibly more. I know I do!
4. Going to a movie theater	Take your own low-calorie popcorn in that adorable oversized purse you just bought. Just make sure you recognize the ingredients on the bag before buying it.
5. Going to happy hour	Skip mixed drinks and opt for a glass of red wine. Or a simple vodka and club soda with fresh fruit (lemon or lime) as a garnish. Drink two glasses of water before ordering an alcoholic refill.

Potential High-Risk Event	Quick Coping Response
6. You just ate two bites of chocolate cake and feel you cannot stop	Quickly pour salt on the cake, or pepper or water—whatever you have handy that can ruin it before you decide to take another bite. Trust me, you'll thank me later.
7. Going to a party or an event in which there is only alcohol to drink and high-fat foods to eat	Hold a drink (could be alcoholic or not) in one hand most of the time. This makes it much harder to eat with the other! And make a plan by setting goals for yourself while you're there. "I will have one glass of wine." Be intentional.
8. Attending a meeting where there is food and you don't want to dig in	Carry breath freshener with you and take a spritz. Or, if possible, go brush your teeth. Who wants to eat when you can taste that minty fresh breath?
9. Home alone with nothing to do	Call a friend, take a relaxing bath, or go for a walk. Consult your list of coping behaviors.
10. You're craving an addictive food and you can't get the taste or image out of your mind	First, be mindful. Notice the urge to eat. Don't judge it; don't try to push it away. Just admit it's there. Now, refocus on an image of yourself as a healthier person who has met her goals.
11. Watching television	Take up a hobby that keeps your hands busy while you watch, such as knitting or doing a jigsaw puzzle.
12. Someone pushes your buttons and you explode with anger	Take a deep breath and focus on something pleasant and beautiful in your immediate environment—a painting, a color, a vase of flowers. Concentrate on that beauty and breathe it in. Allow the beauty to slow you down. Inhale the beauty, exhale the anger.
13. Taking the kids out for ice cream and wanting some, too	If you can't get the feeling to pass, practice harm reduction. Order a low-fat yogurt or sorbet—small and in a cup. No cone!

Potential High-Risk Event	Quick Coping Response
14. Coming home late from work with no time to think about preparing dinner	Consult your list of "go-to" restaurants with your healthy options already picked out. You've made the list in advance for this reason. Now you can make a quick and healthy decision.
15. There are three family picnics this summer that you must attend and you know the food that will be there is all the high-fat food you love	Be assertive and offer to take charge of the menu and insist that there be healthy options that you will plan and bring. Summer flows with fresh fruits and vegetables. There are so many options—put a deliciously positive spin on it.
16. Going away for a special weekend to a beautiful inn with a fabulous restaurant	Keep on food journaling. It's extra important. Write yourself a coping statement: "This weekend is about relaxing with my spouse. It's not all about food."
17. Grazing while Mom makes the holiday turkey dinner	Say you want to pitch in and help prepare the meal. Let her know you want to give your hands something to do other than put food in your mouth.
18. It's been raining or been too cold for 2 weeks and you haven't been able to get outside to walk; your weight loss has plateaued	Head to the nearest mall and do several laps—no window-shopping. Get in extra steps at the supermarket by taking two laps before and at the end of shopping.
19. You get a frustrating e-mail from your boss and find yourself in front of the fridge when you get home from work	Stop. Cope. Choose. Stop: What led me to the fridge in this moment? Cope: Recite a coping statement: "I'm really frustrated right now, but eating that giant bar of chocolate won't take the frustration of the e-mail away." Choose: I am going to choose one small square of this chocolate, put the rest back, and walk into the other room.
20. Discovering there isn't a gym at your vacation site to help you keep up your fitness routine	Consult the Internet, Pinterest, or other sites that offer free at-home workouts. Download a few and don't make excuses!

HOPE FOR THE HOLIDAYS

More famous, or infamous, than the "freshman 15" is holiday weight gain. I've been counseling people with weight problems and food addictions for more than a decade, and I have yet to encounter someone who volunteers to do something about their weight just *before* the holidays. It's the classic mental trap of a chronic dieter: "The diet starts again in January." Bad, bad idea, which brings me to Brain-Powered Pointer No. 31:

Your Resistant Biology never takes a holiday.

After all, you might think, who *doesn't* gain weight over the holidays? Well, here's the honest answer: Most people don't. Research shows the typical holiday weight gain among normal-weight people is only about 1 pound. When I reveal this well-researched fact to clients, I usually get a silent, stunned-face stare in response. Many people who struggle with weight loss see holiday weight gain almost as a universal given, the season of the sanctioned splurge. But this is only because they've been conditioned to think this way.

For many people, it starts with the food-heavy Thanksgiving weekend and the sentimental feasting with family and friends—"It just feels so right." Some start to feel themselves unravel when they put out the crock of candy for Halloween trick-or-treaters ("I try but I can't stop myself from putting my hand in too."). For most of them, it can cause a 5- to 10-pound weight gain, enough to move up another size and bring on the disillusionment that goes with it. This doesn't happen by intention; nobody *wants* to gain weight. It happens because that voice in your head is leading you astray.

If you have a weight problem, there is no doubt that the holidays are a vulnerable time. Your Resistant Biology is working overtime to please your fat cells, and your emotional connection to food is tested by nostalgia, family, and, let's face it, stress. However, here's food for thought: Think about how wonderful it would feel if you stepped on the scale on the first of January and saw what most people see—just a pound or two of damage. Or, better yet, you didn't gain anything at all! So let's get you there by powering your mind for a win-win holiday season.

Monitor, monitor, monitor. A study published in *Health Psychology Research* showed that Long-Term Weight Controllers who self-monitored their behavior during the holidays with cognitive therapy practices like the ones in this book were more successful at managing their weight than a similar group of people who did not self-monitor. Another study found that people who consistently self-monitored for at least 75 percent of the time during the holiday season actually continued to *lose* weight. This means that everything you're learning in this book cannot take a holiday. If anything, you need to intensify what you practice.

Be mindful about your biology. It's rule number one for the holidays. Your Resistant Biology doesn't know it's the holiday season and it doesn't care. When it comes to the caloric impact on your biology, there is no difference between Thanksgiving or Christmas and a day in the middle of June. It isn't going to cut you a break just because everybody else is overeating, but the consequences are much more devastating for people prone to gaining weight, no matter how hard they try to avoid it.

This was proven in a study that compared the effort to resist holiday weight

College Bound? Try This Behavior

Here's a simple behavioral antidote to freshman weight gain: a digital bathroom scale.

Two separate studies conducted at Cornell University wanted to find out if daily weighing would be a useful tool in preventing what has become known as the "freshman 15"—the tendency to gain weight after going off to college.

In both studies, a group of female freshman college students were given a digital scale and told to weigh themselves each morning after getting out of bed. Another group of similar students was given no instructions. After the first semester, the young women in the first study who did not monitor their weight gained an average of 8 pounds. The women in the second study who did not weigh themselves gained an average of 5 pounds. The vigilant scale watchers in both studies gained virtually nothing!

The reason this strategy works lies in its accountability. Just knowing you'll be stepping on a scale in the morning can deter you from choosing the mac 'n' cheese and opting for the grilled chicken instead. Use this strategy only if you feel like the scale works for you, not against you.

gain in two groups of people: Long-Term Weight Controllers (LTWCs) and normal-weight people who have never needed to diet. While the LTWCs worked harder exercising and watching what they ate, they were more vulnerable to weight gain during the holidays than people without a weight problem. Nearly 40 percent of the LTWCs gained 2 or more pounds compared to only 17 percent of the normal-weight people. They also found it more difficult to get rid of the weight after the holidays were over. After 1 month back on their usual schedule, only 10 percent of the LTWCs managed to get back to their preholiday weight.

This is why you must stay acutely aware of every bite you take during the holidays if you want to avoid weight gain. Take the normal amount of food that you are now used to serving yourself and stop when you are satiated. Ask yourself, "What's the point in eating until I'm bulging? Do I really want to feel that way?" Remember, your Resistant Biology takes no holidays. What you overeat is going to find its way to your fat cells. Monitor those calories and stay vigilant with your food journaling.

Be mindful about your choices. With each holiday party and meal you attend, be mindful about what and how much you eat. Consider what you now know about the difference between hunger and desire as well as what you know about your personal triggers. Then ask yourself these questions:

- Am I hungry, or does the food just look good to me?
- What can I do to get away from the buffet table and get my mind off the food?
- When I do make a food choice, what choice will I make that is most in line with my goals?

Catch yourself in the act. When you're at a party with a plate of food in your lap or find yourself on the verge of going for a second helping even though you don't need it, pause and say to yourself: "At any point in time, I can stop the chain of mindless eating. Where am I right now in this chain?" Firm your resolve and walk away.

Try a little aversion therapy—a lot. Don't overeat just because the food is there. Remind yourself how physically uncomfortable it is to overeat, what it feels like when your clothes are too tight, how deflating it is trying to pull up a zipper that doesn't want to budge. Picture an oil slick on top of that eggnog or ants in the fruitcake—whatever will turn you off to something you'd rather not have. Before you put that piece of red velvet cake on your plate, remind yourself how you'll feel emotionally after you eat it. Do whatever it takes to make an off-plan food choice less desirable in favor of a healthier choice or no choice at all. When you wake up the next morning, you'll be thankful you did.

Keep yourself moving. A lot of people get time off around the holidays, so it is an opportunity to get in even more exercise than usual. Take your visiting family or friends to a park or trail they've never been to and do some postmeal walking. Organize a touch football game before turkey time. Getting extra movement in around mealtime will not only stimulate your metabolism for the extra calories you might consume, but also boost your mood and lower your stress levels. One study of overweight men and women found that exercise alone did not protect against holiday weight gain. You have to move *and* monitor your food intake.

Write yourself a holiday affirmation. You know when your time of holiday vulnerability begins, so count back 3 months on your calendar from that date. Write yourself an affirmation that goes something like this: "This year I will not sabotage myself by overeating over the holidays. This year I will continue forward every single day toward my goal of Healthy Obsession." Use this space to write your own or do so in your journal or notebook:

_____

_____

_____

_____

Say it aloud every morning in the mirror until after the New Year. Remember, affirmations can produce extraordinary mind-altering results, and studies show the benefits can be long lasting.

Take portion control to a different level. There is so much variety on that buffet table, and it looks so good you want to taste it all. Well, you can as long as you understand the definition of *taste* as a bite. Ignore the serving spoon and pick up a teaspoon and take it from dish to dish. However, if you're the type of person who can't eat just one cookie or one potato chip, this tip is not for you. Which brings me to my final point.

Find what works for you. I have an office lined with diet books filled with advice on how to keep your diet intact through the holidays: Eat before you go to the party, don't eat standing up, eat from a salad plate rather than a dinner plate, and on and on. The truth about these tactics is that some of these things might work for some people some of the time, but they don't work for all people all of the time. Me? I can tell you that if I eat before I go to a party, I'm still going to eat at the party. If I don't eat standing up, I am certain I won't eat any less once I sit down.

KNOW THAT FOOD

At the Airport

What choice produces the least damage when you get to the airport for an early morning flight and find you only have a few options for breakfast?

- A New York–style bagel smeared with cream cheese
- A glazed doughnut
- A fast-food breakfast egg and cheese muffin
- A Snickers bar from the vending machine

Surprise! You'll find the least amount of calories and fat in the Snickers: 250 calories and 12 grams of fat, compared to 310 calories and 13 grams of fat for the muffin sandwich, 420 calories and 17 grams for the cream cheese and bagel, and 490 calories and 9 grams of fat for the doughnut. However, it's your *worst* choice because it also has 27 grams of sugar, way too much for breakfast or any meal. It will give you a sugar spike that will not only encourage fat storage but will leave you hungry before you get to your destination. The better among these options: The breakfast muffin, as the egg and cheese offer fill-you-up protein and fat and a modest amount of calories.

Your best option is to bring your own food to eat at the airport and on the plane. Pick a protein bar with no added sugar, even two if you need it. Or stock your carry-on with a piece of string cheese, a small handful of almonds, and a pear in a paper bag (remember those?) and you'll have a well-rounded breakfast with protein, fat, and natural sugars that your body will digest in a timely fashion, keeping you full your entire flight.

Airports have notoriously poor choices for weight controllers, making them high-risk situations because they can catch you off guard. Don't let it happen. I learned this a long time ago, and I never travel without an emergency supply of healthy snacks in my carry-on.

So, don't fall for these traps. The only thing that works is what works *for you*. The holidays are a trap for virtually all weight controllers. As individuals, we all have our own triggers and behavior patterns that lure us to eat. You know yours—you worked on discovering them in Step 3. Keep them foremost in your mind when you go through this chapter's key exercise, "Prep Think for High-Risk Scenarios" on page 190.

As for myself, these are my go-to tricks based on my personal triggers and behaviors around foods during the holiday season:

1. I never keep holiday cookies or candy in the house—ever. If somebody gives them to me, I give them away. The reason? I am not good with temptation. I don't need or want to eat them. I know they aren't going to serve me in any way, so I don't want to keep them in my house.

2. When I go to a holiday celebration, I remind myself that food is just fuel. I don't need more at a party than I would at any other time.

3. If I decide to eat something that is not in line with my goals, I mindfully acknowledge that decision and take two or three bites. That's all. I also don't berate myself for tasting something off my plan. I just enjoy and move on.

WHEN STRESS HAPPENS

High-risk situations come in two varieties: those you can anticipate and therefore prepare for (the holidays, the parties, the cruise, whatever), and those that hit us by surprise (a serious illness in the family) or blindside us (being downsized out of your job). "Lose weight, eat healthy with all this stress? Are you kidding me?"

When the curveballs come your way, the best you can do is continue on with the tools you have learned, making every effort to make mindful decisions along the way and take it one day at a time and, when necessary, one step at a time. It's not that you will never lose your grounding—you will. The reality is, when the going gets tough, you can only live in the moment. You can only control what is occurring at a single moment in time.

Throughout this book, you have been building positive cognition patterns, which will become valuable to you in times of crisis—helpful reinforcements that you didn't have before. You've learned, or are learning, to shed the cognitive distortions that drove you to overeat, especially during troubling times. You are now aware of the control you have over your cognitive patterns: "Here's what I can control."

Accept your current situation for what it is, nonjudgmentally, and let the rest go. Recognize that there are still parts of life you can control: "I still can control what I eat." And that is a good thing. While all the world may feel like it's falling apart around you, two things you can control are your thought processes and your eating pattern, and you now possess the tools to make them both positive. Another thing you can work on is building your stress tolerance.

Become an A-A-A-A Advocate

Too much day-to-day stress can insert a lot of skips and bumps in life and make your weight-loss journey feel particularly arduous. You can change the level of stress in your life by enlisting the stress management tool known as the four A's: avoid, alter, adapt, and accept.

Avoid. We unintentionally bring a lot of stress into our lives because we are not mindful of how and why stress enters. Often, it happens because we overextend ourselves. Here are things you can do:

- Learn to say no in the same assertive and firm way you learned on page 188. If you don't want to go to your nephew's Little League

---

Resilience Technique: Learn to Relax

Your emotions are in turmoil and you're tied up in a body knot. Untie it by taking a time-out to do this visualization technique called progressive relaxation, a two-step method in which you first tense, then relax, muscle groups. It is proven to help alleviate emotional stress and anxiety. Some people hold a lot of tension in their bodies without even realizing they are doing it. This will help you bring awareness to those sensations and release them.

If possible, find a quiet place and take about 15 minutes to do this exercise.

Imagine that your body is all tied up in knots and only you know how to untie them. Beginning with your toes, tense your muscles for a few seconds, then relax them. Gradually move your way up your body to your shoulders, then down through your arms to your fingertips. Tense, then relax, each muscle group. As you tense, visualize yourself tightening the knots. As you release, picture yourself undoing them. Repeat two times.

game—"It's so-o-o-o boring"—just say you aren't going. There is no need to make up an excuse.

- Intentionally stay out of the way of people who irritate you and set your goals off balance. If it's someone at work, go out of your way, if necessary, to put physical distance between the two of you, even if you have to ask for a change of cubicle or office.

- Always feeling overextended? Prioritize your day by making a to-do list in order of importance. Do what's at the top, and if you don't have time for it all, let the rest slide.

Alter. Is something going on or about to happen that will annoy you and stress you out? Small problems and irritations turn into bigger ones if they aren't resolved. Take action to change a situation for the better as soon as you see it's taking a wrong path. Communicate your feelings openly and without placing blame—"I feel our team will do the best job possible with a longer deadline."

Adapt. The perception that you can't cope is stressful in itself. Be willing to adapt your own standards and expectations in order to defuse what is leading up to a stressful situation. Enlist these techniques:

- Affirm to yourself that "I can handle this." Say it aloud, over and over, until you believe it.

- Stop negative thinking. When you refuse to assess a stressful situation as being negative, it may cease to be. Instead, reframe it. If there is a 100 percent chance it's going to rain over your ski weekend, then look at it as an opportunity to unwind, read a good book, and enjoy the mountain scenery.

Accept. There will be times when you have no choice but to accept the way things are. You can make acceptance easier without an infusion of stress by doing the following:

- Talk it out with someone in your support group or a friend who can empathize.

- Enlist this affirmation: "I am resilient and will make it through this."

- If you don't like the outcome to a situation, consider it a lesson learned and move on.

Your Stress Buffer Shield

Even though there is never a way to completely prepare yourself for an emergency, you can help build your stress tolerance with what I call the Stress Buffer Shield. This exercise can take some time, and you need to be in a stress-free frame of mind to do it. You do not have to do this exercise now, but you should do it sometime soon, before an emergency strikes, so you have it prepared in your time of need.

Go to a quiet place where you can think and relax. Give yourself all the time necessary to think about the statements. You can go to my Web site, www.elizakingsford.com, and download the document "Stress Buffer Shield" and put it in your notebook or journal, or fill it in below.

Life experiences that have strengthened me and taught me to manage (for example: the death of a loved one):

_____

_____

_____

_____

_____

_____

_____

_____

_____

My support network, the people who nurture and console me:

_____

_____

_____

_____

_____

_____

_____

_____

_____

Attitudes and beliefs that help protect me or help me view things differently (for example: while I know things are hard now, I always have a way of finding my way through a tough situation):

_____

_____

_____

_____

_____

_____

_____

_____

_____

_____

Physical self-care habits that prepare me or help me release tension (for example: I love to walk when I'm feeling overwhelmed; the fresh air seems to clear my thoughts):

_____

_____

_____

_____

_____

_____

_____

_____

_____

Action skills and behaviors I will engage in during stressful times that will support my goals (for example: I will let Amy know when I am struggling and ask for the support I need to get me through this tough time):

_____

_____

_____

_____

_____

_____

_____

_____

_____

_____

Becoming a Long-Term Weight Controller, as you now know, is all about mental preparedness and having the ability to stay in control of a situation in your most capable way—by mindfully directing your thoughts and behaviors, even when they are seemingly out of control. "I can only do the best that I can do." . . . "The only moment I can control is the present moment." . . . "My eating is something I always have the ability to control." . . . "The option is totally mine." . . . When your mind naturally steers in this direction, you'll know you're on your way to crossing the bridge to Healthy Obsession. In the next Step, you'll discover what you can expect once you get there.

META MENTORING WITH ELIZA

His Job Puts Him at High Risk for Eating Too Much

Jim B. is a gregarious and outgoing fellow, the perfect personality for someone who has to attract clients to his money management firm. A big part of his job in wooing wealthy clients is entertaining them, mostly at high-end restaurants or taking them to major league sports events, both of which involve lavish meals. When I first met Jim, he was carrying a good 60 pounds extra on his 6-foot-2 frame and feeling miserable about it. He went to the gym when he could make it, mostly about 3 days a week. The gym offered him a great way to de-stress but was doing nothing to help him lose weight. We pick up the conversation where Jim is describing his typical business-lunch day.

Jim: On the days I know I'm going out for a client lunch, I usually skip breakfast or maybe, if I'm really hungry, I'll eat some pretzels that I keep in my desk. No fat in them, you know. Lunch is usually at a steak house. I order large to make my clients comfortable—appetizers, steak, salads, sides, wine, the works. Besides, I'm a hungry guy. When I get home at night, my wife has dinner ready for the family. I'm not really all that hungry, but somehow I manage to eat what she serves. Got to be a good role model for the kids, you know.

Me: So, what it sounds like you're telling me is that you're starving yourself through the morning so you can overeat at lunch?

Jim: Well, not really. I'm saying I'm trying to save calories by not eating breakfast, because I know I'm going to be eating a lot of calories at lunch.

Me: So, why can't you eat a normal breakfast and a normal lunch and still entertain clients?

Jim (looking at me as if I have two heads)**:** Because I'm entertaining. That's what I have to do. I have to be magnanimous. Order large. Show our appreciation.

Me: So, hold on a second. Let's do a little fact-checking here. Who says that's what you have to do?

Jim: Well, no one says. It's just what you do. My boss expects me to come back with a big expense report. It's what we do.

Me: So, do you think you'll lose your clients if you order fish and a salad and let your clients order for themselves?

Jim: I think it would make everyone feel awkward. Too boring.

Me: Really? How do you know? What's happening is that you're allowing a lot of cognitive distortions to drive your decisions. I see it all the time in situations just like yours. People are on expense accounts, and it's permission to eat too much. People are being entertained, and it's permission to eat too much. Hey, it's a free lunch, so why not order big! The only problem is your Resistant Biology is never going to allow you to overeat without risking the consequences—ever.

Jim (sheepishly)**:** So, that's why I skip the breakfast.

Me: And you arrive at lunch *really* hungry, so you over-order. You're probably over-ordering for everybody.

Jim: You got me there.

Me: How about trying this. Next lunch, eat your breakfast as usual. Go to your steak house, if you'd like, and order a lunch that's in line with your goals—a petite steak or seafood and a salad. A steak house is actually a good choice for a weight controller, because the menu is usually large with a large variety, including a selection of fish, and mostly everything is a la carte. You can order around the menu, if you like, rather than an entrée. Invite your guests to order for themselves. They might actually prefer it. And you can still be magnanimous by ordering a variety of side dishes—salads and veggies—for the table. Try a few low-calorie shrimp cocktail appetizers. That will help fill the table and give you a party atmosphere, if that's what makes you feel comfortable.

Jim: I'll think about it, okay? The other thing is getting home at night. Sometimes these lunches go to 3 p.m., and I really am not all that hungry. But my wife has dinner on the table at 6 p.m. for the kids. It's usually pasta or chicken, stuff they like. Normally it works for me and is in line with my goals, but not on top of a big lunch.

Me: You don't have to be a role model at the dinner table every night. On the days you entertain, let your wife know in advance that you're going to be fixing yourself a tuna salad when you get home. What if being a role model meant being able to say, "I had a big lunch and am not very hungry, so I think I'll stick with just the vegetables tonight." Think about it this way. It isn't really role modeling if you're teaching your kids about overeating.

Next time I saw Jim, he told me he did what I asked and it worked out just fine—"superb" was his word. What surprised him the most was that his clients also ordered seafood, and nobody really bothered much with the extras he ordered for the table. "When I said I was watching my weight, the other guys said they were, too. I guess these kind of lunches can take a toll on everybody."

Cross the Bridge
to Healthy Obsession

*Healthy Obsession: A preoccupation with the planning and
execution of target behaviors used to reach a healthy goal*

You have learned what the planning and execution looks like. You have
learned what your target behaviors look like. You are ready to live a life of
Healthy Obsession.

It's the new you—who you are and where you want to be for the rest of your
life! It can happen when you reach your healthy weight goal, it can happen
while you're on your weight-loss journey, or it can happen weeks or even
months into your new healthy lifestyle. You'll know when it's happening
because you'll begin to realize you no longer struggle to live a healthy life—
you *desire* to live healthy. It's what's making you thrive.

This doesn't mean that you'll never struggle, but it means your inner
power to maintain all you have achieved is greater than your Resistant Biology
and other forces that tempt you to stray. You know you are a weight controller.
You accept it. You recognize it as a work of ongoing progress, a life of vigilance
that's become second nature. You are mindful of your food choices and make
them *after* considering the consequences and rewards. When something goes
awry—"Oh no, I'm up 2 pounds"—you know what to do next. The exercises
you've learned automatically play in your head. You continually tell yourself,
"The present moment is the only thing I can control." You're living a life of
Healthy Obsession, and you relish it. It can be calming. It can be exhilarating.
It can be both. However it feels to you, it is your own personal award.

Healthy Obsession does not make you perfect and it does not mean you can
never ever have a piece of kielbasa or a Milky Way again. It means you now
crave less and less of the foods that caused your weight gain and desire more of

the kinds of foods that serve you. It means you know instinctively what you can eat and how you must exercise to stay there. It means the old self-defeatist tape that caused you to gain weight is in remission—you fall back on it by default less and less. However, you also know you can't allow yourself to become complacent. Non-vigilance is an open invitation to revisit the old you, which brings me to Brain-Powered Pointer No. 32:

You have to use your past to propel your future.

To this end, you must plan for your future by letting go of, but never forgetting, the past. You, the successful weight controller, will forever have a different profile than people who lose weight and eventually gain it back. Studies from the National Weight Control Registry, which tracks people who have lost at least 30 pounds and kept it off for at least 1 year, as well as the records we keep at Wellspring, show a dramatic difference between the two. People who maintain their weight loss say they:

- Consistently monitor their weight control behaviors.
- Keep a close eye on the quality of calories they eat, with an eye on sugar and fat.
- Embrace the need for high levels of physical activity through some kind of aerobic exercise.
- View daily movement as the only acceptable way to get through the day.
- Continue to stay accountable to their daily food intake and energy output through a tracking device.
- Weigh themselves regularly.

In fact, studies comparing LTWCs to people who regained found that weight controllers and weight gainers ate almost the same number of calories day in and day out; the difference was not significant. The researchers concluded that the difference was that the LTWCs consistently continued to manage their behaviors around food and activity. They made healthier food choices and engaged in a more active lifestyle. This means that what you've learned in *Brain-Powered Weight Loss* can succeed for you. It's the last and only weight management program you'll ever need.

A DAY IN THE LIFE OF HEALTHY OBSESSION

Having a Healthy Obsession is exhilarating. When you eat healthy day to day, you wake up each morning feeling more in control of your life. You feel energized. You feel positive. You feel good in your skin. It doesn't mean life is perfect—hardly. It doesn't mean you don't have bad days, disappointments, or even meltdowns. But it does mean that you don't get rattled like you did in the past when stress or a bad break drove you to eat. This is because you have the mental tools to handle it better. You instinctively know that the present moment is the only thing you can control. So, you take a deep breath, put on your Stress Buffer Shield, and pull out the Dealing Skills you've found work best for you.

When you have a Healthy Obsession, your circumstances in life are not all that different, but your view of the world is. Your sense of self-efficacy is different. You know you have the ability to navigate your surroundings in a way that serves you. Healthy Obsession means different things to different people, but those who possess it share one commonality: They handle life as best they can in a way that doesn't sabotage their commitment to their healthy lifestyle. I can't imagine living any other way. Here's a glimpse at what a day in the life of Healthy Obsession looks like, using myself as an example.

I live in Boulder, Colorado, one of the healthiest places on the planet and a wonderful place for an active outdoor life. I have a wonderful husband who shares my enthusiasm for active living and a terrific preschool-age daughter who does more than her share to help keep us on the move. But even with a stage set for an awesome active lifestyle, I know that when I am not living in my Healthy Obsession, I am not living my most authentic life. For me, my Healthy Obsession means that I make choices every day about my food and how I'm going to move my body. And here's the thing: These choices *bring me joy!* They don't feel like a burden or a source of stress for me; they make me feel peaceful. When I am not making conscious decisions about my food and movement, I know I am not at my best.

I wake up with intentions for my day. Even with a toddler who often comes into my room to start my day, I take the time to set my intentions. I will mentally run through what my day looks like. Do I have what I need in the way of food in my fridge? If not, do I have the time to go to the grocery store? If not, what is my plan? This is a quick and automatic process, and it sets me up for success with my food right away. I do the same thing with exercise. How many meetings do I have today? What is my time frame for exercise? When do I plan on getting my movement in? Again, I set myself up for success with intention, rather than letting the day get away from me and hoping I can fit it all in. That is my Healthy Obsession talking.

There are many days when things don't go as planned—an unexpected meeting comes up at work, things take longer than I thought they would, perhaps I am tired. In these cases, I use my Dealing Skills to adjust on the fly. What is in my control? What, if anything, can I change? I remind myself, "I always have a choice," so even if my day fills up and I can't get any movement in and I don't get to the grocery store and I don't have healthy options for food in my house, I always have a choice. If I slow down, get mindful, and use my Dealing Skills, there is always a choice to be made in line with my Healthy Obsession.

Even on the hardest days, the ones that lead to me making a decision not in line with my goals, I know that the measure of my success is always about the next decision I make. I can choose to continue down a path that leads me to feeling frustration, lethargy, and disappointment, or I can choose to not let that decision derail me. Living with my Healthy Obsession day to day has made it automatic that I choose to get right back on track. My Healthy Obsession brings me joy, peace, and a sense of stability with my health. I once heard somewhere, "I am the CEO of my own health." Living with my Healthy Obsession makes me feel like I am in charge of my health each and every day.

LOOKING AHEAD TO
LONG-TERM WEIGHT CONTROL

One of the most important things you can keep in mind moving forward is that losing weight is not the end of a long struggle; it is the beginning of a healthier and more promising life—a new commencement in your life. In order to become a Long-Term Weight Controller, you will want to continue the practices you adopted that make you accountable to yourself:

- Tracking your food intake

- Committing to walking 10,000 (or more) steps a day

- Putting more activity in your life through exercise and intentional movement

- Being mindful of your eating choices, recognizing both the consequence and reward of each decision

- Preventing a lapse from becoming a relapse

- Making and living by daily goals

To keep your commitment, make a contract with yourself, your pledge to maintain a healthy weight and live a healthy lifestyle. It need not be elaborate. In fact, the shorter and more to-the-point you are, the easier it will be to memorize and keep in the front of your mind. Write it down and make it the wallpaper on your computer or a message reminder on your phone. It can go something like this:

I am a weight controller and I accept it. I recognize that my Resistant Biology never takes a vacation and I accept it. I understand that cognitive distortions created the emotions that caused me to turn to food. I vow to not relive my past of overweight and maintain my Healthy Obsession going forward.

Write your own contract to yourself in your journal or the space below, or download the document "Contract to Self" from my Web site, www.elizakingsford.com, for your notebook.

Contract to Self

_____

_____

_____

_____

THE BEST YOU CAN DO IS . . .

Life is never perfect. You know that, I know that. No matter how bad a day may turn out—you feel you couldn't get anything right, you skipped the gym, you ate really poorly, you yelled at the kids and took it out on the dog—at the very least, follow through with my final Brain-Powered Pointer, No. 33:

Don't chalk up any day as a total loss.

There will be times when the best you can do is to be flexible. Do the best that you can do. Never write off an entire day, especially one that started out as a real disaster ("I never should have gotten out of bed today!"). At times like this, it's more important than ever to check in with your goals and look for steps, however small they may be, that will keep you honest to them in some way ("At least I can go out for a quick walk.").

Be mindful. Accept life in the moment on life's terms. See it with clarity. There is no use resisting what you cannot change. There is no sense in taking a bad day and looking for a circumstance or person, especially yourself, to place the blame. Resist doing this, because it is only negative thinking that can bring you to the brink of defaulting to old cognitive distortions and turning to food for self-soothing. Remind yourself, "The current moment is the only one I can control." Remind yourself, "I am a healthy person. I am doing my best." Remind yourself, "I am not taking this lapse into a relapse." When you know you are doing the best that you can do in the moment, there is no need for excuses.

Quite often, when I meet with clients for the last time and welcome them to their life of Healthy Obsession, I give them a copy of my favorite inspirational sayings from the 1997 bestseller, *The Four Agreements* by Don Miguel Ruiz:

Be impeccable with your words. Avoid using words that speak ill of yourself or others. Speak with integrity, using the power of words to direct truth and love.

Don't make assumptions. Find the courage to express your thoughts and ask questions. Communicate with others as clearly as you can to express your needs and feelings. As Ruiz says, "With this one agreement, you can completely transform your life."

Don't take anything personally. Never think that actions others take are because of you. They are merely projecting *their* own reality. "When you are immune to the opinions and actions of others," he writes, "you won't be victim of needless suffering."

And my favorite . . .

Always do your best. Doing your best is all you can do, and it can change from moment to moment. As Ruiz writes, "Under any circumstance, simply do your best, and you will avoid self-judgment, self-abuse, and regret."

It all makes a life of Healthy Obsession self-empowering and totally rewarding. Once you have it, you'll never want to let it go.

ACKNOWLEDGMENTS

There are so many people who helped make this dream a reality for me. My gratitude could never be expressed in a few short "thank yous," but I will try.

To Brad Lamm, without whom this book would never have come to life, thank you for seeing the light in me and encouraging me to share it. To Ryan Craig, thank you for always believing in me. To Debora Yost, thank you for helping me turn my stream of thought into words on paper; you are brilliant. To my terrific agent, Jane von Mehren, thank you for seeing the vision and taking a chance on me. To Mikey Glazer, thank you for always having my back! To the entire Rodale publishing team, especially Marisa Vigilante, Jennifer Levesque, Izzy Hughes, and Gail Gonzales, thank you for being the perfect home for this book.

To my incredible mentors, supporters, colleagues, and friends at RiverMend Health, thank you for your unwavering support and belief in me.

To all the incredible clients, families, and campers that I have had the pleasure of working with over the last 10 years, I am humbled by the opportunity to serve you and to hear your heartfelt stories. I do not take this responsibility lightly. Thank you for your openness and courage. You have taught me more than any book ever will.

To my village of family and friends who have watched me fall off the cliff and disappear into writing, only to welcome me back with open arms, thank you for being my support system. I could not do this life without you.

To my little girl, Quinn, you are the light in my eyes. You make me want to be a better person every single day. I hope I am making you proud.

And most importantly, thank you to my partner, my rock, my husband, Tom. You have been my biggest cheerleader, my fierce companion, and my foundation. You are constantly challenging me to go farther than I think I can go, which is exactly why I love you so dearly.

SELECTED REFERENCES

Abel, M. L., et al. "Consumer Understanding of Calorie Labeling: A Healthy Monday E-mail and Text Message Intervention." *Health Promotion Practice* 16, no. 2 (March 2015): 236–43.

Ahima, R. S. "Revisiting Leptin's Role in Obesity and Weight Loss." *Journal of Clinical Investigation* 118, no. 7 (July 2008): 2380–83.

Arch, J. J., et al. "Enjoying Food without Caloric Cost: The Impact of Brief Mindfulness on Laboratory Eating Outcomes." *Behaviour Research and Therapy* 79 (April 2016): 23–34.

Avena, N. M., et al. "Further Developments in the Neurobiology of Food and Addiction: Update on the State of the Science." *Nutrition* 28, no. 4 (April 2012): 341–43.

Avena, N. M., and M. S. Gold. "Food and Addiction—Sugars, Fats and Hedonic Overeating." *Addiction* 106, no. 7 (July 2011): 1214–15.

Blechert, J., et al. "To Eat or not to Eat: Effects of Food Availability on Reward System Activity during Food Picture Viewing." *Appetite* 99 (April 1, 2016): 254–61.

Blumenthal, D. M., and M. S. Gold. "Neurobiology of Food Addiction." *Current Opinion in Clinical Nutrition and Metabolic Care* 13, no. 4 (July 2010): 359–65.

Boutelle, K. N., et al. "How Can Obese Weight Controllers Minimize Weight Gain during the High Risk Holiday Season? By Self-Monitoring Very Consistently." *Health Psychology* 18, no. 4 (July 1999): 364–68.

Bremer, A. A., M. Mietus-Snyder, and R. H. Lustig. "Toward a Unifying Hypothesis of Metabolic Syndrome." *Pediatrics* 129, no. 3 (March 2012): 557–70.

Brownell, Kelly D., and Mark S. Gold. *Food and Addiction: A Comprehensive Handbook*. Oxford; New York: Oxford University Press, 2012.

Butryn, M. L., et al. "Consistent Self-Monitoring of Weight: A Key Component of Successful Weight Loss Maintenance." *Obesity* 15, no. 12 (December 2007): 3091–96.

Camilleri, G. M., et al. "Association between Mindfulness and Weight Status in a General Population from the NutriNet-Santé Study." *PLOS One* 10, no. 6 (June 3, 2015): e0127447.

Dalen, J., et al. "Pilot Study: Mindful Eating and Living (MEAL): Weight, Eating Behavior, and Psychological Outcomes Associated with a Mindfulness-Based Intervention for People with Obesity." *Complementary Therapies in Medicine* 18, no. 6 (December 2010): 260–64.

D'Arrigo, T. "A Trimmer You. The Right Choices. How to Keep Those Holiday Pounds at Bay." *Diabetes Forecast* 60, no. 12 (November 2007): 32.

Davis, C., et al. "Evidence That 'Food Addiction' Is a Valid Phenotype of Obesity." *Appetite* 57, no. 3 (December 2011): 711–17.

Dietrich, A., et al. "Brain Regulation of Food Craving: Relationships with Weight Status and Eating Behavior." *International Journal of Obesity* 40, no. 6 (June 2016): 982–89.

Dimeff, Linda A., and Kelly Koerner. *Dialectical Behavior Therapy in Clinical Practice: Applications across Disorders and Settings*. New York: Guilford Press, 2007.

Fairburn, Christopher G. *Cognitive Behavior Therapy and Eating Disorders*. New York: Guilford Press, 2008.

Fraser, R., et al. "Cortisol Effects on Body Mass, Blood Pressure, and Cholesterol in the General Population." *Hypertension* 33, no. 6 (June 1999): 1364–68.

Gearhardt, A. N., W. R. Carbin, and K. D. Brownell. "Development of the Yale Food Addiction Scale Version 2.0." *Psychology of Addictive Behaviors* 30, no. 1 (February 2016): 113–21.

Germer, Christopher K., Ronald D. Siegel, and Paul R. Fulton, eds. *Mindfulness and Psychotherapy*. 2nd ed. New York: Guilford Press, 2013.

Godsey, J. "The Role of Mindfulness Based Interventions in the Treatment of Obesity and Eating Disorders: An Integrative Review." *Complementary Therapies in Medicine* 21, no. 4 (August 2013): 430–39.

Gold, Mark S., ed. *Eating Disorders, Overeating, and Pathological Attachment to Food: Independent or Addictive Disorders?* Binghamton, NY: Haworth Medical Press, 2004.

Greenberg, A. S., and M. S. Obin. "Obesity and the Role of Adipose Tissue in Inflammation and Metabolism." *American Journal of Clinical Nutrition* 83, no. S2 (February 2006): S461–S465.

Greenberger, Dennis, and Christine A. Padesky. *Mind Over Mood: Change How You Feel by Changing the Way You Think*. 2nd ed. New York: Guilford Press, 2016.

Holzel, B. K., et al. "Mindfulness Practice Leads to Increases in Regional Brain Gray Matter Density." *Psychiatry Research* 191, no. 1 (January 30, 2011): 36–43.

Karam, J. H. "Obesity: Fat Cells—Not Fat People." *Western Journal of Medicine* 130, no. 2 (February 1979): 128–32.

Katterman, S. N., et al. "Mindfulness Meditation as an Intervention for Binge Eating, Emotional Eating, and Weight Loss: A Systematic Review." *Eating Behaviors* 15, no. 2 (April 2014): 197–204.

Klem, M. L., et al. "A Descriptive Study of Individuals Successful at Long-Term Maintenance of Substantial Weight Loss." *American Journal of Clinical Nutrition* 66, no. 2 (August 1997): 239–46.

Klem, M. L., et al. "Does Weight Loss Maintenance Become Easier over Time?" *Obesity Research* 8, no. 6 (September 2000): 438–44.

Klok, M. D., S. Jakobsdottir, and M. L. Drent. "The Role of Leptin and Ghrelin in the Regulation of Food Intake and Body Weight in Humans: A Review." *Obesity Reviews* 8, no. 1 (January 2007): 21–34.

Leahy, Robert L. *Cognitive Therapy Techniques: A Practitioner's Guide*. New York: Guilford Press, 2003.

Levitsky, D. A., et al. "Monitoring Weight Daily Blocks the Freshman Weight Gain: A Model for Combating the Epidemic of Obesity." *International Journal of Obesity* 30, no. 6 (June 2006): 1003–10.

Linehan, Marsha M. *Skills Training Manual for Treating Borderline Personality Disorder*. New York: Guilford Press, 1993.

MacLean, P. S., et al. "NIH Working Group Report: Innovative Research to Improve Maintenance of Weight Loss." *Obesity* 23, no. 1 (January 2015): 7–15.

Mantzios, M., and J. Wilson. "Mindfulness, Eating Behaviours, and Obesity: A Review and Reflection on Current Findings." *Current Obesity Reports* 4, no. 1 (March 2015): 141–46.

Mason, A. E., et al. "Reduced Reward-Driven Eating Accounts for the Impact of a Mindfulness-Based Diet and Exercise Intervention on Weight Loss: Data from the SHINE Randomized Controlled Trial." *Appetite* 100 (May 1, 2016): 86–93.

McGuire, M. T., et al. "Long-Term Maintenance of Weight Loss: Do People Who Lose Weight through Various Weight Loss Methods Use Different Behaviors to Maintain Their Weight?" *International Journal of Obesity and Related Metabolic Disorders* 22, no. 6 (June 1998): 572–77.

McGuire, M. T., et al. "What Predicts Weight Regain in a Group of Successful Weight Losers?" *Journal of Consulting and Clinical Psychology* 67, no. 2 (April 1999): 177–85.

McKay, Matthew, Jeffrey C. Wood, and Jeffrey Brantley. *The Dialectical Behavior Therapy Skills Workbook: Practical DBT Exercises for Learning Mindfulness, Interpersonal Effectiveness, Emotion Regulation & Distress Tolerance.* Oakland, CA: New Harbinger Publications, 2007.

Mead, N. L., and V. M. Patrick. "The Taming of Desire: Unspecific Postponement Reduces Desire for and Consumption of Postponed Temptations." *Journal of Personality and Social Psychology* 110, no. 1 (January 2016): 20–35.

Neumark-Sztainer, D., et al. "Self-Weighing in Adolescents: Helpful or Harmful? Longitudinal Associations with Body Weight Changes and Disordered Eating." *Journal of Adolescent Health* 39, no. 6 (December 2006): 811–18.

Ochner, C. N., et al. "Treating Obesity Seriously: When Recommendations for Lifestyle Change Confront Biological Adaptations." *The Lancet. Diabetes & Endocrinology* 3, no. 4 (April 2015): 232–34.

Olsen, K. L., and C. F. Emery. "Mindfulness and Weight Loss: A Systematic Review." *Psychosomatic Medicine* 77, no. 1 (January 2015): 59–67.

Pearl, R. L., et al. "Exposure to Weight-Stigmatizing Media: Effects on Exercise Intentions, Motivation, and Behavior." *Journal of Health Communication* 20, no. 9 (2015): 1004–13.

Perito, E. R., L. A. Rodriguez, and R. H. Lustig. "Dietary Treatment of Nonalcoholic Steatohepatitis." *Current Opinion in Gastroenterology* 29, no. 2 (March 2013): 170–76.

Perri, M. G., et al. "Comparative Effectiveness of Three Doses of Weight-Loss Counseling: Two-Year Findings from the Rural LITE Trial." *Obesity* 22, no. 11 (November 2014): 2293–300.

Phelan, S., et al. "Holiday Weight Management by Successful Weight Losers and Normal Weight Individuals." *Journal of Consulting and Clinical Psychology* 76, no. 3 (June 2008): 442–48.

Pomeranz, J. L., and K. D. Brownell. "Can Government Regulate Portion Sizes?" *New England Journal of Medicine* 371, no. 21 (November 20, 2014): 1956–58.

Pope, L., et al. "New Year's Res-illusions: Food Shopping in the New Year Competes with Healthy Intentions." *PLOS One* 9, no. 12 (December 16, 2014): e110561.

Roberts, S. B., and J. Mayer. "Holiday Weight Gain: Fact or Fiction?" *Nutrition Reviews* 58, no. 12 (December 2000): 378–79.

Schoeller, D. A. "The Effect of Holiday Weight Gain on Body Weight." *Physiology & Behavior* 134 (July 2014;134): 66–69.

Schulte, E. M., N. M. Avena, and A. N. Gearhardt. "Which Foods May Be Addictive? The Roles of Processing, Fat Content, and Glycemic Load." *PLOS One* 10, no. 2 (February 18, 2015): e0117959.

Shriner R., and M. Gold. "Food Addiction: An Evolving Nonlinear Science." *Nutrients* 6, no. 11 (Nov. 21, 2014): 5370–91.

Stevenson, J. L., et al. "Effects of Exercise during the Holiday Season on Changes in Body Weight, Body Composition and Blood Pressure." *European Journal of Clinical Nutrition* 67, no. 9 (September 2013): 944–49.

Trust for America's Health and the Robert Wood Johnson Foundation. *The State of Obesity: Better Policies for a Healthier America 2014.* http://healthyamericans.org/assets/files/ TFAH-2014-ObesityReport%20FINAL.pdf.

Wagner, D. R., J. N. Larson, and H. Wengreen. "Weight and Body Composition Change over a Six-Week Holiday Period." *Eating and Weight Disorders* 17, no. 1 (March 2012): e54–56.

Wing, R. R., and S. Phelan. "Long-Term Weight Loss Maintenance." *American Journal of Clinical Nutrition* 82, no. S1 (July 2005): S222–S225.

Yanovski, J. A., et al. "A Prospective Study of Holiday Weight Gain." *New England Journal of Medicine* 342, no. 12 (March 23, 2000): 861–67.

INDEX OF EXERCISES
AND WORKSHEETS

INDEX

Underscored page references indicate sidebars and tables. **Boldface** references indicate illustrations.